Ethics in Nursing Practice

ETHICS IN NURSING PRACTICE

Basic Principles and
their Application

F. J. Fitzpatrick

The Linacre Centre
for the Study of the Ethics of Health Care

London 1988

Published by the Linacre Centre, 60 Grove End Road, London NW8 9NH.

First published 1988.

British Library Cataloguing in Publication Data

    Fitzpatrick, F. J.
    Ethics in Nursing Practice: basic
    principles and their application
    1. Medicine. Nursing. Ethical aspects.
    I. Title. II. Linacre Centre.
    174'.2

    ISBN 0-906561-05-1

Typeset by MFK Typesetting Ltd., Hitchin, Herts.
Printed and bound by Redwood Burn Ltd., Trowbridge, Wilts.

To the memory of
Sister M. Xavier O'Donnell

Devoted Religious and distinguished nurse educator

CONTENTS

FOREWORD

The Linacre Centre was established in May 1977 as a research and education centre in the field of health care ethics. Our principal goal is that of providing intellectual support to fellow Catholics engaged in clinical and allied work to enable them to maintain and develop in that work a commitment to the characteristic values of their moral tradition.

The Governors and staff of the Centre were made aware at an early stage in our existence of the need for a comprehensive account of nursing ethics which would be both faithful to Catholic moral tradition and accessible to a wider audience. The need for a general text was urged upon us not only by individual nurses but also by representatives of the Guild of Catholic Nurses and the Association of Nursing Religious.

Because of other commitments of our small staff it was not possible to begin to address this need until 1984, when Dr. F. J. Fitzpatrick joined the Centre staff. It was decided to entrust to him the task of preparing a general text on nursing ethics. In this work Dr. Fitzpatrick has had the benefit of generous advice from a small group of nurses and nurse educationalists who have met from time to time at the Centre to discuss his drafts. Responsibility for the text rests, however, with Dr. Fitzpatrick.

The Centre is very grateful to him for the contribution he has made to its educational programme in the present work. *Ethics in Nursing Practice: Basic Principles and their Application* seeks to expound an approach to nursing ethics which is faithful to the Catholic tradition, while at the same time making clear the profoundly reasonable defence of human dignity – the dignity of the nurse and the dignity of the patient – which that tradition stands for. In these tasks of exposition and clarification Dr. Fitzpatrick has drawn on his considerable training as a philosopher.

Ethics in Nursing Practice is not an easy read. It invites nurses to think hard about the values, the attitudes and the principles which should inform their professional work. The challenge it poses is one which will surely be widely welcomed by all who recognise the independent character of nursing as a profession, and the responsibility the profession therefore has to maintain in our confused times a sound ethical basis for its commitment to the care of patients.

Sir John Dewhurst FRCOG, FRCSE
Chairman of the Board of Governors, The Linacre Centre

INTRODUCTION

Among the most difficult moral problems faced by people in the course of their work are those which arise for health professionals. To say this is not to suggest that people in other walks of life rarely have to face pressing moral difficulties, for this is clearly not the case. But since medical and nursing work typically involves treating people who are in a debilitated and vulnerable condition, and whose very lives are often at stake, the moral problems raised by contemporary medical and nursing practice are especially urgent. For a long time those who investigate and discuss ethical problems in health care have tended to concentrate largely on problems arising for doctors, while taking little note of the difficult issues faced by nurses in their day-to-day work. This imbalance is decidedly odd, because nurses are typically more, not less, immersed in the care of their patients than are doctors – a nurse is with her patients more or less constantly while she is on duty, whereas a doctor's consultations may often last only a couple of minutes – and the crucial decisions which have to be made by nurses on hospital wards are, surely, every bit as difficult and demanding of careful thought as those faced by a doctor. I suspect that what lies behind this lopsided emphasis on doctors' problems is the feeling, often unexpressed but powerfully at work in the background, that nurses' problems just are doctors' problems, admittedly experienced from a slightly different angle, but not containing anything new of substance. On this view it would be a waste of time to write a book devoted specifically to ethical problems arising in nursing, because such a book would merely amount to a text of medical ethics slanted, to some extent, toward the nurse's point of view. Such an attitude naturally goes hand-in-hand with the idea that the sum-total of a nurse's activity consists in carrying out treatments prescribed by a doctor, and that she performs her work well to the extent that she provides these treatments satisfactorily, badly to the extent that she fails to do so. There is, on this view, no specifically nursing activity, distinct from that of the doctor, which requires skill and understanding and which can give rise to difficult moral issues.

The idea that nurses' problems are really doctors' problems, although seen from the standpoint of the one carrying out orders rather than the one issuing them has in the past been widespread. But it is nevertheless clearly false, as I argue in Chapter One of this book. There is a great deal more to nursing than the carrying-out of medical treatments, and in some fields of nursing, such as health visiting and care for chronically- and terminally-ill patients, there may in any case be very little in the way of medical treatment to carry out. There are, then, genuine nursing activities which are distinct from medical work; and this means that there are ethical problems arising in nursing which differ from those arising in medicine. Hence, a serious consideration of ethical problems raised by nursing practice is by no means a superfluous activity, and the fact that problems of nursing ethics have been much discussed in books and articles over the past few years is testimony to a greatly increased awareness of this fact.

Anyone who seriously considers the sorts of ethical problems which can confront nurses is bound to be struck by the sheer range and variety of these problems, as well as by their intellectual difficulty. There can be no question of stating, investigating and resolving these problems in a brief compass, and so we find that recently-published books on nursing ethics tend to be fairly sizeable volumes, without, for all that, managing to cover anything like the full range of ethical difficulties which can arise. The present volume inevitably suffers from these limitations. I have outlined and defended a basic account of what morality and moral reasoning are all about and applied that account to various representative problems arising in nursing practice. But I cannot claim either that the general approach to morality defended here is discussed in the detail which it deserves – that would require a far more lengthy investigation than is possible here – or that anything like an exhaustive range of moral problems has been discussed. Although I have argued that many difficult moral problems in nursing have definite answers, that there are actions which are, in themselves, morally right and others which are morally wrong, the point of this book is not to lay down answers to the various problems treated but rather to help nurses themselves to think through these problems in a way which consistently respects genuine moral requirements.

The conviction that there *are* such things as "genuine moral requirements", that morality is not a matter of our personal subjective opinions but of objective truth, is one of the features of a natural-law approach to ethical issues which sets it apart from many popular conceptions of morality today. The natural-law approach to ethics has been closely associated with the teaching office of the Catholic Church. But an important part of this approach has been the claim that in principle, many important ethical truths can be seen to be true without any reliance on divine revelation or Christian tradition. There may be disagreements over the question of how far this ability extends, with some natural-law moralists claiming that *all* moral truths knowable by human beings can be apprehended solely on the basis of unaided human reasoning, but others replying that certain moral truths need to be based specifically on Christian teachings. I suspect that the attempt to justify *all* ethical beliefs on a purely natural basis is misguided, and that (for example) the idea that man has an inherent dignity which requires to be respected is unjustifiable except on the view that man is a being "made in the image and likeness of God", as the scriptures tell us (Genesis 1, 27). However this may be, it has been my aim in writing this book to avoid, as far as possible, appeals to specifically Christian teaching, although I have often referred to such teaching for illustrative purposes. Again, while my primary concern has been that of helping the Catholic nurse to approach and handle intelligently the moral problems which are likely to come her way, I hope that the emphasis laid in this book on philosophical argument and on the moral "data" which can be apprehended by all people without any explicit appeal to specifically religious teachings will enable it to be helpful to the non-Catholic or non-Christian reader. The nursing problems discussed here, and the general theoretical and moral questions which need to be answered first before the nursing problems can be dealt with fruitfully, are admittedly difficult: I have tried to write about these questions and problems with as much clarity as I can achieve, in the hope that even the complex philosophical considerations which are occasionally dwelt on at length are discussed in such a way that the reader without any special training in philosophy will be able to follow them.

In the course of writing this book I have accumulated a number of debts which I now take pleasure in acknowledging. The Director of the Linacre Centre, Mr. Luke Gormally, has been a keen and penetrating critic of successive drafts of this work; his criticisms are all the more appreciated by me in that his own administrative and research duties have been so onerous and time-consuming. Members of the consultative committee set up by the Linacre Centre to oversee production of the manuscript were also generous with their help, which was particularly important to me because they were able to contribute that knowledge of and familiarity with nursing "from the inside" which was so valuable in guiding my steps through the complex problems posed by modern nursing. One of the members of this consultative committee was Sister Xavier O'Donnell, Senior Tutor Emeritus in the Nightingale School of Nursing at St.

Thomas's Hospital, London, and a governor of the Linacre Centre, who died suddenly in March this year and to whose memory this book is dedicated. While researching for and writing this book I was able to talk over regularly with Sister Xavier various aspects of the problems dealt with here, and benefited greatly from her breadth of knowledge and long experience as a nurse and nurse tutor, and particularly her keen awareness of the importance of the concepts of professional responsibility and accountability for nurses today. Her death deprived the Linacre Centre of a very able and generous supporter. With Sister Xavier on the consultative committee were Mr. Stanley Holder, Miss Bernadette O'Farrell, Miss Ellen Perry and Professor Penny Prophit, who contributed much to the task of clarifying my ideas and pointing out where they failed to take full account of the complexity and professional character of modern nursing. In naming these people I cannot, of course, presume to imply their agreement with everything that I say in this book; on the contrary, I am solely responsible for the views expressed here and for mistakes which are made. This same proviso applies, of course, in the case of those other people whose generous help I must acknowledge, particularly Mr. Iain Colquhoun, Dr. John Finnis, Mr. Tom Keighley, Miss Mary McLaughlin, Mrs. Agneta Sutton and Miss Carolynn Williams, all of whom commented on drafts of various chapters or particular arguments which I was proposing. Special thanks are due to my wife Mary, whose keen interest in the issues examined here and strong support for my labours in tackling them has been a great help to me from beginning to end.

F.J.F.
25 August, 1988.

CHAPTER ONE

NURSES, THE NURSING PROFESSION AND ETHICAL PROBLEMS

How should a nurse face up to the ethical problems which she encounters in her work? In trying to decide what action to take, how should she analyze the problems she is facing so as to identify the moral issues at stake? Questions of this sort will be central to the investigation of this book. In order to begin getting to grips with them, let us consider a problem of a kind which arises frequently for nurses in hospital wards. The problem, as expressed by a nurse at a London teaching hospital, is as follows:

> "It is often difficult to answer the questions of patients who have just had a cancer diagnosed. In many cases they are not told the severity of the disease or the prognosis, and nurses are not supposed to tell them if the doctor wants the information withheld from them. We at ... Hospital had a patient who came in for tests which disclosed that he had a cancer of the rectum. He was not told of his condition, but was simply informed that he was to have a colostomy. This news quite terrified him. We were not allowed to tell him why he was to have a colostomy, because he was already a nervous man and the doctors considered that the news would affect his condition. Even so, he kept asking us if he had a cancer, and insisting that he would rather know definitely than not know. We told all this to the doctors, but they still refused to inform him."

Likewise, it may happen that at a ward meeting the nurse in charge will state: "Dr. X instructs that Mr. A [a patient] is not to be told about his condition". Any nurse caring for Mr. A would, then, apparently be required not to tell him the truth about his condition but to evade any awkward questions which he may raise. It may even be suggested that the nurse is morally obliged to lie to Mr. A, to tell him, for instance, that he is suffering from some remediable muscular problem when in fact he has motor neurone disease. May a nurse accede to requests of this sort? Or is she obliged to answer the patient's questions truthfully, to tell him what she herself knows about his condition and his prospects?

Some people would suggest that in situations of this sort the nurse's proper course of action is to suppress her own convictions and to do as the doctor says. If the nurse herself thinks in this way, she may reason to herself as follows: "I don't myself think it's a good thing to evade Mr. A's questions, and if it were up to me I should give him the whole truth. But unfortunately it's not up to me. It isn't my place to tell him what he wants to know; it's the doctor's job to do this, and if I were to tell Mr. A the whole truth I'd be usurping the doctor's role. I must be satisfied to do those things which are my own legitimate business and not try to take over responsibilities which belong to other people."

A nurse who thinks in this way is evidently basing her moral judgment on a certain conception of her role precisely as a nurse. What is this conception? It is that of the nurse as essentially the doctor's handmaid, someone whose first loyalty is not to her patient but to the doctor who prescribes medical treatment for the patient: her proper role is precisely that of ensuring that this prescribed treatment is carried out and also of looking after the patient whenever the doctor is not around to attend to him personally.[1]

This conception of what nursing is all about has at times been widely held, by nurses themselves as well as in society at large. Against it, however, there is the view of nursing which finds expression in many of the recently-formulated codes of professional conduct. For instance, the code issued in 1976 by the Royal College of Nursing lays it down that "The primary responsibility of nurses is to protect and enhance the wellbeing and dignity of each individual person in their care".[2] If this is the case, it is arguable that no nurse may decide that she should not tell her patient about his condition simply because the patient's doctor has instructed her not to do so. Here we seem to have two incompatible conceptions of what nursing is and what the nurse should be doing.

These reflexions lead us to draw the following conclusion: this moral problem raised by a doctor's instructions not to tell patients about their

---

[1]   "The first and most helpful criticism I ever received from a doctor", wrote an American nurse, Sarah Dock, in 1917, "was when he told me that I was supposed to be simply an intelligent machine for the purpose of carrying out his orders." (Quoted by M. Benjamin in the *Hastings Center Report*, vol. 18, no. 2, April/May 1988, p. 38.)

[2]   Royal College of Nursing of the United Kingdom, *RCN Code of Professional Conduct – A Discussion Document* (London 1976), p. 1.

conditions or prospects, like many moral problems arising in nursing, can be intelligently handled only if one has first determined what the proper role of the nurse consists in. For in general, people are often morally obliged, by virtue of their filling a certain role in society, to act differently from those who have not assumed that role. A parent, for instance, has obligations towards his children – e.g., to provide for their material well-being and education – which no mere friend of the family could be said to have. Just as someone who becomes a parent thereby incurs a totally new set of obligations, so one who takes on a particular occupation is morally obliged (normally, at least) to perform faithfully the activities which that position entails. In some occupations the employee's responsibilities will have been either exhaustively described to him or enumerated in his contract, so that no detailed inquiry into their nature will be called for. But in other occupations, including nursing, the practical decisions which need to be made may vary enormously from one day to the next, so that no precise enumeration of "dos" and "don'ts" could ever be formulated. We need, then, to become as clear as we can about the proper role of the nurse. There are all kinds of situations in which a nurse who finds herself morally impelled to act in a certain way may hold back, asking herself: "Is it my *place* to do this? Do I, in my position, have the *right* to take the matter into my own hands in this way? Have I the *authority* to do so?" Such questions are essentially questions about the nature of the nurse's legitimate role, and about the sorts of acts and omissions which adherence to that role may license. So at least some of the moral problems which the nurse encounters will be soluble only if she possesses a clear-headed awareness of what is involved in being a nurse.

The role of the nurse

One traditional answer to this question about the nurse's role is that the nurse is engaged in *caring* for people who are either ill or disabled or (as in the case of some pregnant women) who require some fairly close and regular attention if certain dangers to life and health are to be avoided. According to this line of thought, the maintenance of health is a basic human need which people normally meet through eating and exercising, maintaining the right bodily temperature, and so on. This normal method of maintaining health may go wrong in either or both of two ways. First, the activities which normally maintain health and physical well-being may no longer be sufficient to do so. If this happens, because of illness or injury, and if, also, the patient cannot himself make up the difference, some fairly intensive and more or less prolonged caring may be necessary. Secondly, the patient, due to either illness or injury, may no longer be able even to perform those activities of eating and exercise which are essential for health, and in this case also someone else will have to care for him by helping to provide whatever he needs in order to have his health restored and maintained. The activity of helping or caring may require considerable skill and also a detailed knowledge of the workings of the human body, the nature and consequences of the patient's condition and the complications which might arise from it, and so on. This task of caring for a patient, in the effort to maintain him in health or to restore him to health, is that which is proper to the nurse. In the case of those, such as terminally-ill patients, who cannot be restored to full health or anything like it, the nurse's role will be that of assisting the patient to retain (and, if appropriate, to regain) as much of his health and physical well-being as he possibly can, given his condition.

This conception is well summarised in the following account of the nurse's function, taken from one of the best-known general nursing textbooks, Virginia Henderson's *Basic Principles of Nursing Care*:

> The unique function of the nurse is to assist the individual, sick or well, in the performance of those activities contributing to health or its recovery (or to peaceful death) that he would perform unaided if he had the necessary strength, will or knowledge. And to do this in such a way as to help him to gain independence as rapidly as possible. This aspect of her work, this part of her function, she initiates and controls; of this she is master. In addition she helps the patient to carry out the therapeutic plan as initiated by the physician. She also, as a member of a medical team, helps other members, as they in turn help her, to plan and carry out the total programme whether it be for the improvement of health, or the recovery from illness or support in death . . .
>
> . . . the primary responsibility of the nurse is to help the patient with his daily pattern of living, or with those activities that he ordinarily performs without assistance; these are breathing, eating, eliminating, resting, sleeping and moving, cleaning the body and keeping it warm and properly clothed. The nurse also helps to provide for

those activities that make life more than a vegetative process: namely, social intercourse, learning and occupations that are recreational and those that are productive. In other words she helps the patient to maintain or create a health regimen that, were he strong, knowing and filled with the love of life, he would carry out unaided.[1]

How, in this case, does the nurse's role differ from that of the doctor? The answer is that the doctor has special knowledge and skills which enable him to diagnose illnesses, to give prognoses and to prescribe courses of treatment for the acutely ill – that is, for those illnesses which can be treated by radical intervention in the functioning of the body, e.g., by surgery or drugs. He is also able to prescribe similar treatment for the palliation of the symptoms of disease in both the acutely ill and the chronically or terminally ill. The nurse's training does not give her the knowledge and expertise to carry out the first of these tasks, and so in the treatment of acute illness, and in some aspects of the care of the chronically or terminally ill, she helps to implement a programme of treatment prescribed by the patient's physician. Even so, provided that the nurse does, in these cases, faithfully carry out her part in the medical or surgical procedure, the nursing care which she provides is something on which she, and not the patient's physician, is the authority. So, on this view, whereas a doctor's priority is normally the *cure* of illness or disease, or at least the attempt to achieve as much in the way of a cure as can reasonably be hoped for, the nurse is concerned primarily with the *care* of patients. In some cases this nursing care will be used to assist the doctor in his efforts to cure, but in other cases (including, most obviously, those involving terminal illness) it will not.

This amounts to saying that the nurse's role can be seen as encompassing both an *independent* and a *dependent* function. That is, her work comprises both those activities which she performs as an independent practitioner and those other activities which she performs in helping to implement programmes of treatment prescribed by another health professional, usually a doctor. In her independent role, the nurse is concerned to assist and promote the patient's own bodily and mental resources so

---

1. V. Henderson, *Basic Principles of Nursing Care* (Geneva, 1977), pp. 4, 6. See also the account of nursing provided by Baroness MacFarlane of Llandaff and G. Castledine in their *A Guide to the Practice of Nursing Using the Nursing Process* (London, 1982), pp. 4–5.

that he will recover his health to the fullest possible extent. This aspect of the nurse's role is perhaps most prominent in caring for mentally handicapped patients and also in community nursing and health visiting, where she is concerned, above all, not to do things for her patients but to educate and encourage them to promote their own health or the health of those (infants or aged relatives, for example) for whom they are caring. *Promotion of health* is therefore the central focus of the nurse's attention when she acts as an independent practitioner. But in her *dependent* function the nurse adopts, temporarily, the same perspective towards the patient as that of the doctor who prescribed the treatment, and she puts into effect a medical treatment aimed at directly attacking the disorder from which the patient suffers.

The role of the nurse is, then, a complex one, encompassing an independent as well as a dependent function. According to the condition of the patient whom she is treating, one of these two roles will be more prominent than the other. If the patient is acutely ill, his illness or injury will have to be combated before his natural powers of recuperation will be able to assert themselves. So here the nurse's dependent role is to the fore. But once the acute condition has been rectified, the need is for the patient's own natural powers to be brought into play; and here the nurse's independent role becomes crucially important. This is also true in the case of chronic and terminal illness, where radical interventions in the workings of the body often cannot benefit the patient.

This distinction between the nurse's and the doctor's role should not be made too sharp, for the doctor is not concerned solely with counteracting illnesses and infections and repairing damage to the body. He will realize that radical intervention in the workings of the body, through drug therapy, for example, or through surgery, will not be sufficient to restore the patient to health. The most crucial part in bringing about someone's recovery is played not by anything which a doctor prescribes but rather by the patient's own natural bodily resources. Medical and surgical treatment should be seen not as restoring the patient to health, but rather as removing certain severe obstacles to the effective operation of the patient's own natural health-giving powers. The distinction between medical and nursing roles is really one of emphases or priorities. The doctor concentrates his attention on the effectiveness of therapeutic interventions in the workings of the body, but he will realize that such interventions are not going to achieve anything unless the patient's own health-preserving resources are sufficiently powerful to take advantage of them. The nurse, by contrast, makes the patient's natural health-giving resources for preservation of health her central concern; but since she realizes that these resources can often be rendered ineffective by illness and injury, she sees it as part of her role to help in carrying out the medical or surgical treatment of the patient.

This fact of the complexity of the nurse's role may explain why some writers apparently fail to spot any unifying principle in nursing.[1] They tend to focus their attention on the notion of nursing as essentially caring for patients, and then point out that many activities performed by nurses – the administration of chemotherapy, for instance, or the resuscitation of patients undergoing cardiac arrest – are in fact therapeutic interventions in patients' bodies. They also point out that nurses now regularly carry out treatments involving complex monitoring equipment which were previously the exclusive preserve of physicians, and that these treatments are far removed from caring in the traditional sense. These difficulties disappear once we realize that the nurse's role is complex in the way described, that it contains a dependent and also an independent function, so that no one type of activity will exhaust the nurse's role. We may, then, conclude that caring, in the sense described here, is the nurse's central activity, even though her work also encompasses other duties which are related more or less closely to this central function. Given that the nurse is concerned with the health of the whole person, it is understandable that part of her work will overlap with that of the doctor. So, as one commentator points out:

> Nursing is a process through which *care* is provided to individuals, families, or community groups *primarily* around circumstances and situations that arise from health-related problems. Medical practice, on the other hand, is primarily cause- and cure-orientated. It is important in the above definition to stress the word "primarily", for settings, numbers and other circumstances can change the degree of overlapping functions between the nursing and medical professions. For instance, in remote areas nurses often come closer to practising medicine than nursing. Similarly, a physician may sit beside his patient in the recovery room caring for the subtle circumstances that arise during the postoperative course, practising something more akin to nursing than to medicine.[2]

---

[1]   Cf. A. MacIntyre, "To Whom is the Nurse Responsible?", in C. P. Murphy and H. Hunter, *Ethical Problems in the Nurse-Patient Relationship* (Boston, U.S.A., 1983), p. 79.

[2]   S. Chater, *Operation Update: The Search for Rhyme and Reason* (New York, 1976), pp. 5, 6.

A crucially important concept: health

The nurse's role has been described here as centred on enabling the patient to retain or regain health by encouraging and supplementing the workings of his natural powers of self-preservation and recuperation. With this description, have we arrived at a satisfactory account of nursing? No, not quite. For the very notion of *health*, which figures so prominently in the definition, is subject to differing interpretations. According as one adopts one or another of these definitions of health, one will understand the nature of nursing in differing and, indeed, incompatible ways.

The concept of health not an easy one to analyze, and there is an extensive literature in which the claims of various rival definitions are canvassed. In recent times there have been two leading contenders:

(1) The idea of health as essentially *bodily well-being*. According to this conception, the word "health" applies first and foremost to the proper functioning of the human body. Someone is healthy if his body is functioning as it should, free from disease and injury and from such other impediments as excessive fat levels, muscular flabbiness, high blood pressure and so on. The idea is not that a person is healthy only if his body is functioning *perfectly*, for if this were the case no-one at all, probably, would ever be healthy. Health is well-functioning, not perfect-functioning: it consists in an "all-round satisfactory performance" of the body as a whole and of its individual parts and organs.

Supporters of this definition of health as bodily well-being do not deny that it makes sense to say that someone is healthy in mind as well as in body; nor do they dispute that a person's mental and emotional state often strongly influences, for good or ill, his physical condition. But they do maintain, first, that the primary use of the adjective "healthy" is to apply to living bodies, and secondly that although health professionals must take account of their patients' states of mind in planning their medical treatment or nursing care, the fact remains that mental and emotional influences on health are just that: factors which profoundly influence health one way or the other but are not actually part of a healthy or unhealthy constitution. I shall call this conception "the somatic conception of health" (from the Greek word *soma*, meaning "body").[1]

---

[1] This conception of health, which dates back at least to Aristotle (384–322 B.C.), is defended in Leon Kass's article "Regarding the End of Medicine and the Pursuit of Health", in A. L. Caplan, H. T. Engelhardt and J. J. McCartney (eds.), *Concepts of Health and Disease: Interdisciplinary Perspectives* (Reading, U.S.A., 1981), pp. 3–30.

(2) The definition of health proposed by the World Health Organization, in its *Constitution* of 1946, as "a state of complete physical, mental and social well-being". On this view, everything which contributes to the good of man is the legitimate business of the health professional. I shall call this "the all-encompassing conception of health".[1]

Those who reject the somatic conception contend that it involves regarding the patient as *just* a body, an organism made up of working parts, and not a human person. They may then object that any health professional who adopts such a conception may easily be led to "depersonalize" his patients, to think of (and perhaps even treat) them as objects rather than people. But this objection evidently involves a misunderstanding. The nurse who accepts the somatic account of health will certainly guide her actions towards patients by her understanding of what will truly promote their physical well-being. But this is not to say that she ignores her patients' personal qualities and treats them throughout as mindless bodies or automata. Her professional concern is with their physical well-being; but she knows that wherever there is a living human body there is a human *person*, and that the body is not an entity in its own right but rather a "part" or aspect of the whole person. She realizes, then, that the point of all her activity is not to serve the body *as such*, but to serve the whole human being through promoting one important aspect of his total well-being, that of health. Admittedly, there is always a danger that health professionals will overlook their patients' individual and spiritual qualities and treat them merely as systems of physical organs; but the somatic conception of health cannot justly be charged with licensing that wrong outlook.

It might be thought that the definition of health as bodily well-being is undermined by the fact that we can speak meaningfully of people being healthy in mind as well as in body, about the mental health of patients, and about certain health professionals, such as psychiatrists and psychiatric nurses, being concerned primarily with mental rather than physical health. This objection is not conclusive, however, because a defender of

---

[1]   The W.H.O.'s definition reads, in full: "Health is a state of complete physical, mental and social well-being and not merely the absence of disease or infirmity." This definition is the first of a series of principles which are stated in the Constitution and which, the W.H.O. declares, "are basic to the happiness, harmonious relations and security of all peoples." (The W.H.O. Constitution is reprinted in Caplan, Engelhardt and McCartney, *Concepts of Health and Disease*, pp. 83–4.)

the somatic conception can say that although the primary meaning of "health" is "bodily well-being", nevertheless the meaning of the word can be extended to cover man's mental functioning. Further extensions in the meaning of the word will make it intelligible to talk of the economic health of a nation, the moral health of an individual or society, the healthy or unhealthy state of a man's spiritual life, and so on. Mental health is, then, on this view, conceived as the harmonious well-functioning of the mind, corresponding to the well-functioning of the body which is health in the strict sense of the word. The fact that it makes perfectly good sense to say of someone "He's mentally disturbed, but so far this hasn't undermined his health" indicates that one is justified in viewing bodily well-being as what is primarily signified by the word "health".

What, then, of the role of psychiatrists and psychiatric nurses? As health professionals their concern is obviously with health; but since it is mental, not bodily, well-being which they are trying to promote, their activities would appear to provide a living disproof of the somatic theory. Is this really the case? What makes this question difficult to handle is the fact that the status of psychiatry itself is a matter of dispute, so much so that either or both premises on which this argument against the somatic theory rests – (1) that psychiatrists *are* health professionals and nothing other than that, and (2) that psychiatry focuses its attention specifically on the patient's mental well-being – are questionable. A behaviourist psychologist, for instance, would certainly challenge the second of these contentions, since he would refuse to recognize any such thing as specifically mental health. If we reject behaviourism and insist that the psychiatrist indeed deals with mental, not physical, well-being, this will be precisely a ground for saying that he is not concerned with the *health* of his patients, in the strict sense of the word "health", and that he should not be regarded as a health professional. It has indeed been the accepted practice for psychiatrists to be medical practitioners, but one may doubt whether this is at all necessary; perhaps psychologists or others could do this work just as well. One could go on to argue that the work of the psychiatric nurse is implicated in this uncertainty surrounding that of the psychiatrist, and that insofar as she concerns herself expressly with the mental well-being of her patients, she is no longer focussing on their health, in the strict and primary sense of this word, and so is moving beyond the field of nursing as such. On this view, psychiatric nursing would be a sort of hybrid occupation, involving nursing *and* some other kind of work which is expressly focussed on patients' mental well-being. This is one possible response which the somatic theorist may take. I do not wish to defend this or any other conception of psychiatric nursing here, but simply to point out that since the status of psychiatry and psychiatric nursing are subject to some dispute, it would seem unreasonable to overthrow our conviction that health in the primary sense is bodily well-being, and that health professionals are those whose attention is focussed primarily on the promotion of bodily well-being.

It can, however, be objected that the somatic account is too vague to be of much use, because the notion of bodily well-being is itself in need of clarification and cannot therefore be used to define health. What, after all, is bodily well-being? How do we measure it? To what extent, if at all, is it compatible with various illnesses and injuries? Is the standard of bodily well-being the same for all men, or does it vary from one person to another, or for different people in different societies? And can we define bodily well-being without first defining the opposed concepts of illness and disease? Clearly any attempt to defend the somatic conception of health by resolving these questions would involve developing a full account of human nature. It would have to be shown that all human beings do possess a common nature, and that the workings of man's body can correctly be described in a *teleological* way, as intrinsically geared to achieving an end or goal (Greek *telos*, "end"), this goal being the bodily well-functioning which the somatic theorist takes to be identical with health. This sort of argument would be far too complex to be conducted here; but much valuable work in this area has been done, and it would be rash to claim that adherents of the somatic conception of health are unable to answer the sorts of question posed above.[1]

What about the all-encompassing definition of health proposed by the World Health Organization? This definition does seem to be open to serious objection. If health is really "a state of complete physical, mental and social well-being", and if the nurse's role is to promote the patient's health, then there are no obvious bounds to the nurse's professional competence and responsibility, or, therefore, to her professional authority. She will embody in her person the roles of social worker,

---

[1] Cf. Kass, *art. cit.*, and also Kass's "Teleology and Darwin's *The Origin of Species*: Beyond Chance and Necessity?", in S. F. Spicker, ed., *Organism, Medicine and Metaphysics* (Dordrecht, 1978), pp. 97–120. Cf. also the remarks of J. J. Haldane in "'Medical ethics' – an alternative approach", in *Journal of Medical Ethics*, vol. 12, no. 3, Sept. 1986, pp. 145–150.

psychologist and priest or spiritual advisor. But this, surely, is unreasonable. It is one thing to say that since the nurse's patients are human persons she must, in caring for them, take account of their mental and spiritual qualities; but it is quite another thing to claim that the patients' spiritual welfare (say) comes under her direct professional competence or that her advice and orders in that field have any professional authority. The nurse's competence and authority have definite limits, and she would act wrongly in attempting to usurp the roles of social workers and chaplains.

A comparison with the role of another kind of professional, a bank manager, may be helpful here. Any bank manager who regarded his customers solely as depositors and borrowers of money and who, in his dealings with them, never took account of their personal and spiritual qualities would certainly be adopting a wrong attitude towards them. He should, instead, fully respect his customers as human persons and deal with their problems sympathetically, as befits human beings. Given that financial problems can impose a severe strain on families, it is probably not uncommon for a manager's attitude to be decisive in (for example) either sustaining a marriage or contributing to its break-up. But to say this is not to say that the bank manager's professional competence is all-encompassing, that he has a direct concern with his customers' personal fulfilment, with the quality of their intellectual, emotional and spiritual lives and with the stability of their marriages. For he *is* a bank manager, not a priest or a marriage counsellor, and his direct professional concern is with those financial matters which his customers entrust to him. It is only insofar as the more intimate aspects of his customers' lives impinge upon their financial position, and *vice versa*, that he can be justified in inquiring into them and offering his customers some limited guidance concerning them.

The question of the nature of health is more complicated than these very brief comments would indicate, and it would be a mistake to imply that the two theories discussed here, the somatic theory and the all-encompassing theory, are the only ones worth examining. On the contrary, there are several other conceptions of health which have been outlined in recent times, and any full treatment of this problem would have to take them into account.

While the reflexions of these pages certainly do not establish the truth of the somatic theory of health – a task which would be impossible in such a brief compass as this – they do, I think, render suspect those theories which seek to go beyond man's bodily well-being and to define health in much broader terms. The least that can be said of the somatic theory is that it is reasonable in itself and that there is no obviously conclusive objection to it.[1]

The account of the role of the nurse which has been reached here is, then, as follows. The nurse's primary aim is that of facilitating the proper functioning of her patients' own resources for preserving and regaining health, to the extent to which that goal is attainable. And the notion of health which is used here is that of bodily well-being, not that of the comprehensive psychosomatic well-being suggested by the World Health Organization. The nurse realizes, of course, that her patients are not just bodies but persons, with mental and spiritual characteristics, and she is concerned to treat them always *as* persons. But her primary focus is on the bodily health which is appropriate to them as living beings. What has just been described is the nurse's primary and independent function; but insofar as her exercising this function leads her to co-operate in administering treatments decided upon by other health professionals she has another, this time dependent, function. However, the dependent function is subordinate to the independent, one, because it is the aim of enabling the patient's health-preserving or health-regaining powers to work unhindered which gives point to all the nurse's activities.

The importance of centring care on patients

Given that the nurse's primary task is to provide care for her patients, it follows that her overriding loyalty is to them. It is important to state this, because the fact that most nurses work in hospitals and spend much of their time in carrying out orders can lead them to mislocate their primary

---

[1.]   Cf. again Kass, "Regarding the End of Medicine and the Pursuit of Health". A recent book, David Seedhouse's *Health: The Foundations for Achievement* (Chichester, 1986) is entirely devoted to this problem. Seedhouse rejects some widely-favoured definitions of health and proposes an alternative definition, according to which "a person's health is equivalent to the state of the set of conditions which fulfil or enable a person to fulfil his or her realistic chosen and biological potentials" (p. 72). This account of health seems to me to be vulnerable to the same objections as those encountered by the W.H.O. definition, *viz*, (1) that it enlarges the scope of health so widely that it would encompass absolutely everything that contributes to man's good, and (2) that it would justify a practically unlimited extension of the doctor's and the nurse's professional competence and authority. One severe weakness of Seedhouse's book is that he does not seem to recognize the somatic theory as one of the theories deserving discussion, and does not refer even once to Kass's important article which outlines and defends that theory.

loyalty. They can come to be preoccupied with satisfying the demands of consultants or of the hospital administration, rather than with responding to the needs of the patients in their care. Admittedly, the opposition between these different viewpoints should not be exaggerated: the well-being of patients provides the *raison d'être* for the work of the hospital administration and the consultants just as it does for nurses; ideally, all three work harmoniously together to achieve a common goal. Nevertheless, administrative procedures in hospitals, as in other institutions, are liable to be seen and pursued as ends in themselves, particularly if a hospital is regarded as a sort of business, with efficient management of staff and resources the number one priority. And hospital consultants, whose personal contact with patients is sometimes minimal, may tend to regard patients as interesting challenges to medical science rather than as whole *persons* whose health problems can be the occasion of profound mental and spiritual suffering. Take, for instance, the following report:

"While working on a male surgical ward I was not at all impressed with the consideration shown by the consultant for patients' feelings. On one particular ward round, he went up to a patient's bed and said loudly: 'Uh, this is the carcinoma, is it?'. As it happened the man was Spanish and spoke very little English, and so probably didn't understand what the consultant had said – which was just as well, because he had only just been admitted and knew nothing of his condition. However, several of the other patients must have heard, and I think this was very thoughtless. Unfortunately this was not an isolated incident, because this particular consultant habitually discussed cases with colleagues in the hearing of patients."

This consultant evidently viewed his patient primarily as a collection of physical organs, one of which was in an interestingly pathological condition. This lack of respect for patients is by no means characteristic of all hospital consultants, because nurses, physiotherapists and others are also capable of treating patients in a degrading manner; but the fact is that nurses, because of their comparatively close relationship with their patients, are normally less inclined to behave in this way. However, the temptation to regard patients not as persons requiring considerate care but as (say) machines to be kept going may nevertheless often be present. All the more reason, then, why the nurse should not allow her attitude to her work to become doctor-centred (or, for that matter, hospital-administration-centred) rather than patient-centred: she must always treat her patients as whole human beings and regard their well-being as the goal of her efforts.

Along with this attitude of overriding concern for the patient's well-being, there are certain qualities of character which appear to be important for any nurse. Her patients – whether she meets them in hospital, in a medical practice or on health-visiting rounds – have genuine health problems which can affect them profoundly on an emotional and spiritual level. A nurse would prove herself insensitive and unfeeling if she were not aware of this fact and able, to some extent, to "enter into" the minds of her patients and appreciate just what their condition means to them personally. Hence the attitudes of concern and compassion, of sensitivity to patients' deepest personal feelings and reactions, should be part of the nurse's conscious make-up.

Two features of current nursing practice can perhaps tempt the nurse to cease regarding her patients as the primary focus of her work and can also weaken her hold on these essential personal qualities. The first of these is the effect of modern technology. Much of a nurse's time nowadays is taken up with operating various pieces of equipment, especially those used in the intensive care of acutely-ill patients. As a result, nurses can come to be absorbed in technological procedures and to regard the areas in which their knowledge and skills are most properly applicable – the continuous care of acutely-ill patients and almost total care of the chronically and terminally ill – as of secondary importance only. One nurse educator reacts to the recent changes in the following way:

> Prior to the miracle drugs and the rapid technological advances in medicine in this century, nursing and its caring functions were the main contributions to health care. The focus was on care of the hopelessly ill individual and not the instant cure of disease. As the practice of medicine became more enhanced in the cure of disease, the quantity and quality of caring on the part of nurses decreased and the nurse became an extension of the physician's technology. The nurse as a medical technician has led to a model of nursing care that is fragmented, dehumanized and depersonalized. Loss of its caring identity and the abandonment of its caring functions has threatened the basic structure of nursing. A return to caring concern now offers hope for the future as nurses begin to value the types of caring services they are capable of rendering to those patients beyond the

reach of medical technology – the chronically ill, the elderly and the terminally ill.[1]

Is this a reasonable reaction to the technological orientation of modern nursing? Arguably it is not, because this technical orientation is an inevitable result of scientific advance and is evidently here to stay. Nurses need to react to these technical changes positively, by trying to handle the demands which they make without relinquishing their patient-centred perspective; they should not react (as, it seems, the author of the quoted passage would recommend) by wishing that the technology would go away and then concentrating on other things. Nevertheless, it certainly is true that the technological character of modern nursing can tempt the nurse to move away from her proper role *vis-a-vis* her patients and to come to see herself instead as a medical technician.

The second factor which can tempt a nurse to abandon a patient-centred perspective has to do with the mode of operation of hospital bureaucracies.[2] Bureaucracies are typically concerned above all with efficiency in achieving the ends for which they are working; but they cannot themselves determine what those ends will be, because the ends are set by other people or bodies, and the bureaucrats take those ends as "givens" which are to be achieved as efficiently as possible. In a pluralistic society like our own, in which there is no public consensus on what sort of a good health is, or how it fits in with the ensemble of other human goods, hospital administrators will lack any coherent conception of the good of health and its place in the achievement of overall human well-being, and will therefore tend to run their hospitals along the same efficiency-conscious lines as any other business. The real end or primary purpose of health-care facilities will tend to be forgotten in the pursuit of efficiency – particularly, of course, money-saving efficiency. Such a policy may powerfully influence nurses working in a hospital or undertaking community nursing for a local health authority; and a nurse whose thoughts are centred on satisfying this demand for efficiency rather than on meeting the needs of her patients will herself be losing sight of the primary purpose of such institutions, with potentially harmful results both for her patients and for herself.

---

[1]   C. P. Murphy, "Models of the Nurse-Patient Relationship", in C. P. Murphy and H. Hunter (eds.), *Ethical Problems in the Nurse-Patient Relationship*, p. 10.
[2]   I am indebted here to an unpublished paper by A. J. L. Gormally, entitled "Risks", which was originally read to a nursing conference in 1984.

The nurse as an advocate on her patients' behalf

The fact that patients, not hospital administrators or other health professionals, are the primary focus of the nurse's activities has led many people to seize on the idea of *advocacy* on behalf of patients as expressing the proper spirit of nursing. The word "advocacy" tends to be given different senses by different writers, and some of these senses are perhaps less appropriate than others; but all those who describe the nurse as "the patient's advocate" hold the following viewpoint. The nurse should, in carrying out her duties, think first and foremost of the welfare of her patients. She should regard herself as an advocate on their behalf, in the sense that she will do everything in her power to obtain for them the care that they need; she will not be afraid to press for their genuine needs to be met if the actions or directives of hospital administrators, doctors or other nurses stand in the way of their being met. In particular, while she will always respect legitimate authority in her hospital, she will not abandon her responsibility to act in her patients' best interests if by so doing she should come into conflict with mistaken directives given by a physician or a nursing superior. This idea seems plainly correct: given that the nurse's labours are orientated first and foremost to the patient's welfare, advocacy on the patient's behalf, in this sense of the word "advocacy", is a duty for her.

Paediatric nurses have recently expressed concern about the possibility that some newborn babies are being admitted to surgery without having been given adequate anaesthesia. According to one advisor to the RCN association of paediatric nursing, "Lots of ward sisters have asked for my support when they've felt that junior medical staff have failed to provide adequate anaesthesia". Another paediatric nurse is reported as saying that "it is now up to nurses to improve their knowledge to guide and advise junior doctors when necessary".[1] Here we have an example of nurses acting as advocates for their patients in a way which is clearly justified – especially since the patients in this case cannot defend their own interests and need someone to advocate on their behalf.

Some nursing writers are inclined to present the nurse as *the* patients' advocate, but this is evidently untenable. For all health professionals, nurses, doctors, physiotherapists and others, should be advocates for their patients, in the sense of "advocate" which is being used here: there is

---

[1]   C. Campbell, "Growing Pains", in *Nursing Times*, vol. 83, no. 43, October 28, 1987, p. 18.

no reason for supposing that nurses monopolize this role. Nevertheless, it does seem that doctors, and especially hospital consultants, because they spend only a short time examining and talking to their patients, may be strongly tempted to treat them in a way which fails to respect their dignity as persons. By contrast, the nurse, who spends much more time in her patients' company, will not normally experience this strong temptation; and in this sense advocacy on behalf of her patients is likely to be a more prominent aspect of her work than of the doctor's.

The nurse-as-advocate viewpoint is sometimes understood as contributing to an adversarial, rather than a co-operative, relationship between nurse and doctor, and there is no doubt that a nurse who takes her role as advocate seriously may sometimes come into conflict with medical personnel. One issue which may generate such a conflict is that of the doctor's duty to obtain informed consent for treatment. If it becomes clear that a doctor has not adequately explained to a patient what his proposed course of treatment will amount to, a nurse may be obliged to intervene in some way so that this unjust situation will be rectified. As one author puts it, "doctors have a legal duty to obtain consent to operations and other procedures and to do so in a manner which ensures validity of that consent." Hence, she goes on,

> If a nurse is aware that consent is being or has been obtained in a manner which invalidates the intention of the law, then there is a clear obligation to make this known to the relevant authority. Failure to do so implicates the nurse in an illegal act...

> [Likewise] Giving information to patients is increasingly accepted as a major role of the nurse, and there is a huge and growing body of research suggesting that information can help patients by reducing stress and by teaching coping strategies, thus reducing pain, the likelihood of complications such as infections and length of stay in hospital... [But] it is not difficult to imagine circumstances in which a nurse giving information like this may cause a patient to question what a doctor has said, or to realise implications which the doctor has not made clear.[1]

But just as there is no reason in principle why advocacy on patients' behalf should be confined to nurses, there is also no reason why it should always

[1]. C. Webb, "Speaking up for Advocacy", in *Nursing Times*, vol. 83, no. 34, August 26, 1987, p. 34.

be directed against the actions or omissions of doctors: for nurses, other health professionals and hospital administrators can act in a way which threatens the genuine well-being of a patient, and a nurse who acts as an advocate for her patient will be concerned to defend the patient against all threats to his integrity and well-being, from whichever quarter they may come.

The nurse as a health professional

In affirming that the nurse has her own proper knowledge and expertise which is independent of (although often employed in order to assist) the doctor, we are in effect affirming that the nurse is a health *professional*, that she belongs to the *profession* of nursing. This fact is commonly accepted, because the phrase "the nursing profession" is in widespread use. But the point of calling the nurse a professional may be unclear, since the word "profession" is difficult to define, and different people understand it in different ways. Here I shall utilize one definition which would command widespread agreement, that given by R. H. Pyne in his *Professional Discipline in Nursing: Theory and Practice*. Pyne sets out seven criteria, all of which must be satisfied by any body which is to count as a profession. They are:

1. Its practice is based on a recognised body of learning which is proper to itself.

2. It establishes an independent body for the collective pursuit of aims and objects related to these criteria.

3. Admission to corporate membership is based on strict standards of competence attested by examinations and assessed experience.

4. It recognises that its practice must be for the benefit of the public and not primarily for that of its practitioners.

5. It recognises its responsibility to advance and extend the body of learning on which it is based.

6. It recognises its responsibility to concern itself with facilities, methods and provision for educating and training future entrants and for enhancing the knowledge of present practitioners.

7. It recognises the need for its members to conform to high standards of ethics and professional conduct set out in a published code with appropriate disciplinary procedures.[1]

Of these criteria, (1) and (7) appear to be the most basic. It is the possession of a body of learning, and concern for proper ethical standards in the application of that body of learning, which are central to the idea of a profession. Criteria (2)–(6) could probably be seen as implications of one or both of these two basic points.

Some social scientists have been reluctant to admit nursing as a profession along with medicine, teaching, law, accountancy, etc., on the grounds that the first criterion is not, after all, satisfied. For, they argue, it is the medical profession which provides the theoretical and practical basis for nursing, and hence the nurse has no advanced knowledge or skills which are proper to her *as a nurse*. But it can be replied that the nurse has a proper role, centred on the provision of care for patients, which is distinct from that of the doctor, that the task of nursing differs from that of medicine, and hence that the knowledge and skills required by nurses will in large part be specifically nursing knowledge and skills. The fact that nurses often use those skills in assisting physicians or surgeons in no way overthrows this conclusion. The contribution of specialist nursing research which is all the time being conducted also tells against this objection: what is being built up here is precisely "a recognised body of learning which is proper" to nursing.

Of the other criteria, (2) and (3) are satisfied by the fact that bodies such as the United Kingdom Central Council for Nursing, Midwifery and Health Visiting exist and operate to promote excellence in nursing. The fourth is satisfied by the actual practice of nurses and by the provisions of the law in respect of their work. The fifth and sixth criteria, as Pyne points out, "while always receiving some attention, have (perhaps) received less attention in the past than was deserved. Happily this has been changing

---

[1] R. H. Pyne, *Professional Discipline in Nursing: Theory and Practice* (Oxford, 1981), pp. 5–6. (I have modified slightly the wording of the first and fourth criteria, in order to make them even more precise than they are in Pyne's book.) Some other writers who set out criteria for professional status allow that not all such criteria need to be satisfied if a body is to count as a profession: "In reality few occupations ever meet all the many criteria, but, to the extent that they do, they can be placed on a scale ranging from most to least professional." (M. S. Pernick, "Medical Professionalism", in *The Encyclopaedia of Bioethics* (New York, 1978), vol. 3, pp. 1028–1034, at p. 1028.)

for the better in recent years as more evidence of valid nursing research has been seen, as the increased membership of nursing and health service staff organisations has led to more articulate and comprehensive expression of concern at any shortfall in both these respects, and as individual nurses have become more aware of the fact that their personal professional responsibility extends into these areas."[1] Finally, the seventh criterion is clearly satisfied, since it is precisely the concern to maintain high ethical standards which explains the disciplinary regulations of the UKCC and similar bodies and which also underlies current debates about crucial problems of nursing ethics in numerous books and nursing journals.

Because nurses work not merely as individuals but as members and representatives of the nursing profession, one of their responsibilities will be to uphold always the standards of the profession, to conduct themselves in a way which observes and respects those standards, and to encourage and assist their fellow nurses to act likewise. It follows that one of the pitfalls faced by nurses will be that of acting in a way which directly betrays those professional standards or condones such action in others. One of the functions of the UKCC and equivalent bodies in other countries is to investigate cases in which it is alleged that a nurse has not observed these standards, cases in which there is thought to be professional misconduct.

While many of the ethical problems which arise in nursing can be discussed without any reference to the idea of the nurse as a health professional, there are some problems in which the professional or unprofessional character of a nurse's action occupies centre stage, so to speak. Much of the opposition to nurses' ever going on strike, for example, is based on the claim that striking is at odds with the nurse's fulfilment of her obligations to her clients and is therefore unprofessional. It is interesting to note that some nurses have considered their professional status incompatible not only with going on strike, but even with engaging in collective bargaining on pay and conditions with employing

---

[1.] Pyne, *Professional Discipline in Nursing*, pp. 6–7. Some writers also see the professional status of nursing reflected in the increasing importance of various specialized nursing roles. Cf., e.g., Monica E. Baly, *Professional Responsibility* (Chichester, 2nd edition, 1984), p. 12: "Another pointer to the growing professionalism of nursing is that it is developing a number of nursing specialisms ... as a response to various medical specialities. Good examples of 'nursing' specialisms are terminal care nursing, stoma therapy and infection control ..."

authorities.[1] This attitude is surely unjustified: given that nurses have to earn their living through nursing, they are entitled to ensure that what they see as just demands for wages and working conditions are brought to their employers' attention. But the very fact that this aversion to collective bargaining has been widespread indicates the strength of the feeling that such action is unprofessional. Some brief attention will be paid to problems concerning industrial action in the final chapter of this book. All that need be said here is that this is an issue to which considerations of the nurse's professional status are highly relevant. In reflecting on issues like this we realize that the idea of the nurse as a professional, as committed to an ideal and a set of professional standards, does have important implications for nursing ethics.

★ ★ ★

This Chapter in Summary

We need to begin by looking at what we might call "the role of the nurse"; for many ethical problems in nursing are soluble only on the basis of an understanding of what the nurse's role or characteristic range of activities is – at least, to the extent that the sheer variety of nursing activities enables that role to be delineated clearly. A commonly-held view has been that the nurse's role is centred on caring for patients, where caring is to be explained as assisting the patient's own health-giving and health-restoring powers to function. This explanation, suitably developed, seems to be satisfactory – provided that it is kept in mind (1) that words like "caring" cannot be defined with any great precision and hence that it may be impossible to mark off the nurse's role from those of other health professionals with absolute clarity, and (2) that an important part of the work of many nurses consists in assisting other health professionals, especially doctors. Since the nurse's work is aimed at promoting the health of patients, it is important to understand health should be defined.

---

[1]   Cf. editorial, "Withdrawal of service – a dilemma for nursing", in *The Canadian Nurse*, July 1968, p. 29: "Although the past few years have brought great changes in attitude among a large portion of the CNA [Canadian Nurses' Association] membership, there still remain many nurses who are reluctant to become involved with collective bargaining to achieve goals. They take a negative attitude toward it, because they believe it to be incompatible with professionalism, or afraid of facing possible conflict with management."

The traditional account of health as bodily well-being seems preferable to more comprehensive definitions such as that of the World Health Organization. Nurses should regard the interests of their patients as vitally important, and contemporary talk of the nurse as an advocate on behalf of her patients has the merit of highlighting this priority. The fact that nurses are members and representatives of the nursing profession is also something which will strongly influence their approach to various ethical problems.

CHAPTER TWO

ETHICAL PROBLEMS IN NURSING: WHAT HELP DO THE PROFESSIONAL CODES GIVE US?

One of the hallmarks of a profession is, as we have seen, the existence of one or more bodies which in a sense govern the conduct of its members. They have two ways of doing this: first, they lay down rules of conduct to which members are expected to adhere at all times; and secondly, they enforce these standards by penalising those who infringe them, the penal sanctions extending as far as withdrawal of a member's licence to practise. Clearly nursing, as practised in Western countries, meets this requirement. In Britain, the United Kingdom Central Council for Nursing, Midwifery and Health Visiting (UKCC) produces a *Code of Professional Conduct*, intended, it says, for "the guidance and advice of all registered nurses, midwives and health visitors"[1]; and the UKCC also operates the disciplinary committee to which those accused of breaching the code are summoned to appear. In addition, the International Council of Nursing in Geneva issues its own code of professional conduct, although this body possesses no disciplinary jurisdiction over nurses in a particular area; and the same is true of the international Catholic nurses' organization CICIAMS, many of whose members also belong to their own national nursing organisations.[2] Codes of professional conduct are documents of considerable importance in nursing today, because they are seen as setting basic standards of practice which nurses must attain. We need, then, to look more closely at some of the nursing codes which are available. The discussion of this chapter will be centred on two questions. First, do the various codes express the same sort of attitude towards nursing and the nurse's role as that expressed in Chapter One of this book? In particular, does the key conception defended in Chapter One – of the nurse as

---

[1] UKCC, *Code of Professional Conduct for the Nurse, Midwife and Health Visitor* (second edition, London, 1984), p. 4.

[2] The letters "CICIAMS" stand for "Comité Internationale Catholique des Infirmiér(e)s et Assistant(e)s Médico-Sociales" (International Catholic Committee of Nurses and Medico-Social Workers).

someone concerned above all for her patients' welfare, and also as committed to co-operating with other health professionals and to maintaining the standing of the nursing profession as a whole – also find expression in the codes? Secondly, to what extent do the professional codes help us in tackling ethical problems in nursing? Is the help which they give significant or only slight? Could it even be claimed that a good code of ethics is *all that a nurse needs* to resolve pressing moral problems?

(1) The codes and the professional role of the nurse

The major conclusions of the last chapter could be summarized as follows:

(i) The nurse should be motivated primarily by a concern to promote the welfare of her patients; she is untrue to her vocation if she is concerned above all with carrying out orders efficiently, or being on good terms with her fellow-workers, etc.

(ii) The nurse is a member of a profession, the nursing profession, which exists in its own right and is not an ancillary service for some other body such as the medical profession. Nursing has its own characteristic range of activities and its own standards of performance which are set by representatives of the profession and not imposed by any outside body.

(iii) Nevertheless, because the patient's health is the nurse's overriding concern, she must work in concert with other health professionals; and this will involve gearing her own activity to (e.g.) courses of treatment prescribed by medical specialists.

(iv) Because of certain features which distinguish nursing from other health-care work – and particularly because of the much greater time which nurses spend with their patients than other health professionals – certain qualities of character are especially appropriate for the nurse: qualities of compassion for those who are ill and vulnerable, of concern for the patient as an individual, of respect for his qualities of temperament and personality, his cultural background and convictions on ethical and religious matters, and so on.

Let us now look briefly at some codes of professional conduct to determine whether all these points find expression there. Clearly the first point, that the nurse works, above all, to promote her patient's welfare, is of primary importance. So we find that the UKCC's code states, in its preamble:

> Each registered nurse, midwife and health visitor shall act, at all times, in such a manner as to justify public trust and confidence, to uphold and enhance the good standing and reputation of the profession, to serve the interests of society, and above all to safeguard the interests of individual patients and clients.[1]

And the first two provisions in the same code specify that nurses are to act on the basis of this patient-orientated perspective:

> Each registered nurse, midwife and health visitor is accountable for his or her practice, and, in the exercise of professional accountability, shall:
>
> 1. Act always in such a way as to promote and safeguard the well-being and interests of patients/clients.
>
> 2. Ensure that no action or omission on his/her part or within his/her sphere of influence is detrimental to the condition or safety of patients/clients.[2]

Likewise, the code published in 1973 by the International Council of Nurses states that "The nurse's primary responsibility is to those people who require nursing care".[3] Of course, the various codes usually go well beyond this statement of overriding principle and specify some ways in which the nurse's concern for her patient is to be translated into action. The UKCC code, for example, states:

> 10. [Each registered nurse, midwife and health visitor ... shall] Have regard to the environment of care and its physical, psychological and social effects on patients/clients, and also to the adequacy of resources, and make known to appropriate persons or authorities

---

[1]. UKCC code, p. 3.
[2]. *Ibid.*
[3]. International Council of Nurses (ICN), *Code for Nurses* (Geneva, 1973), para. 4.

any circumstances which could place patients/clients in jeopardy or which militate against safe standards of practice.[1]

The second and third key conclusions of the last chapter, that nursing is a distinct profession, with its own standards and procedures, and that nurses co-operate freely with other health professionals to benefit patients, is also expressed in the various codes. The UKCC code, for instance, states:

> 5. [Each registered nurse, midwife and health visitor ... shall] work in a collaborative and co-operative manner with other health care professionals and respect their particular contributions within the health care team.[2]

But here too the primary orientation towards the patient's welfare has to be kept in mind. For if someone were to ask: "Why should nurses co-operate with other health professionals?", the answer is that if they do not do this their patients' well-being, and even their lives, could be at risk. The code issued by the Royal College of Nursing in 1976 makes explicit this connexion between co-operation with other health professionals and the overall aim of promoting the patient's welfare:

> In general, relationships with colleagues in nursing and in other health care professions should be determined according to what will maximise the benefit of those in their care.

The gloss on this provision states:

> The goal of 'whole person treatment' determines how nurses should relate professionally to their fellow nurses and to members of other health care professions. It is assumed that the more there is co-operation and communication between the different people caring for the patient, the more the patient's needs are likely to be understood and catered for.[3]

Since nursing is a profession in its own right, for which the maintenance of high standards of care is vitally important, a nurse will be concerned not just with what takes place in her own hospital or clinic but with the

---

[1]. UKCC code, p. 3.
[2]. *Ibid.*
[3]. Royal College of Nursing of the United Kingdom, *RCN Code of Professional Conduct – A Discussion Document* (London: RCN, 1976), p. 3.

standing of the profession as a whole. She will consider it important that correct nursing standards should be adhered to and promoted not only in her own place of work but by nurses generally, and she will want to help to achieve this. Moreover, she will want the profession to be held in high regard by the public, who need to have confidence in the ability and willingness of nurses to strive always for their patients' welfare. The following provisions of the UKCC code can be seen as implying and directly following from these facts concerning the nurse's professional ·status:

[Each registered nurse, midwife and health visitor . . . shall:]

3. Take every reasonable opportunity to maintain and improve professional knowledge and competence.

. . . .

12. In the context of the individual's own knowledge, experience and sphere of authority, assist peers and subordinates to develop professional competence in accordance with their needs . . .

13. Refuse to accept any gift, favour or hospitality which might be interpreted as seeking to exert undue influence to obtain preferential consideration.

14. Avoid the use of professional qualifications in the promotion of commercial products, in order not to compromise the independence of professional judgement on which patients/clients rely.[1]

Provisions (13) and (14), in particular, can be properly understood only against the background of a concern that the profession itself be held in public esteem; for if there were not this concern for the public standing of the profession, why should anyone bother about whether or not (say) a nurse takes part in a television advertisement for some health preparation? The nurse must, then, as the UKCC code states, "act, at all times, in such a manner as to justify public trust and confidence [and] to uphold and enhance the good standing and reputation of the profession . . ."[2]

[1.] UKCC code, pp. 2–3.
[2.] *ibid.*, p. 2.

The last of the four key conclusions of Chapter One is that there are certain attitudes towards patients – most importantly, attitudes of compassion and of respect for patients as individual persons – which are appropriate for nurses. The Canadian Nurses' Association's *Code of Ethics* affirms the appropriateness of these attitudes in the following two "general principles":

> 1. The human person, regardless of race, creed, colour, social class or health status, is of incalculable worth, and commands reverence and respect.

> 2. Human life has a sacred and even mysterious character and its worth is determined not merely by utilitarian concerns.[1]

These two comments are somewhat startling, because they attribute to human beings qualities which would seem to belong to them only on a religious view of man's nature and destiny. For how can man's life be "of incalculable worth", commanding "reverence" and possessing "a sacred and even mysterious character" unless human beings are not chance products of brute physical forces, but, as the Scriptures tell us, "made in the image and likeness of God" and destined by God to a life of intimate fellowship with Himself? In saying this my intention is not, of course, to reject these statements of the Canadian code, but simply to express my suspicion that they are defensible only on specifically religious grounds. However, the principle that the nurse must always respect her patients as individual human beings who are valuable in themselves, and not mere means to be used by others, is stated in all the codes, even if not always with the religious overtones of the CNA's code. The RCN code, for instance, states:

> Discrimination against particular individuals, for whatever reason, should never be tolerated.

And the gloss on this prescription is as follows:

> Entering the nursing profession involves a commitment to the service of persons, each of whom merits individual respect ... the adoption of a professional attitude requires that all those who need nursing care should receive it without discrimination. No group of

---

[1]. *CNA Code of Ethics: An Ethical Basis for Nursing in Canada* (Ottawa, 1980), p. 5.

patients or clients should be regarded as unworthy or undeserving of professional concern.[1]

(2) How far do the codes take us?

All the codes surveyed here proclaim that nursing is a professional activity which is centred on the welfare of individual patients. Once we commit ourselves to this conception of nursing, we can, with the aid of the precisions set out in the various codes, recognize that certain types of behaviour towards a patient are out of keeping with a nurse's proper role and are therefore not to be engaged in. To take an example mentioned in the RCN code, a nurse who deliberately neglects a patient because of his religion or race refuses, in effect, to treat that patient with the respect which belongs to him simply as a human person and therefore acts wrongly. Likewise, consider the following statement and its accompanying gloss, again from the RCN's code:

> Measures which jeopardise the safety of patients, such as unnecessary treatments, hazardous experimental procedures and the withdrawal of professional services during employment disputes, should be actively opposed by the profession as a whole.

> [Gloss:] Actions which betray people's confidence in the professional integrity of nurses diminish the ability of the profession to be of help. For this reason the nursing profession should be clearly seen to be opposed to exploitation of vulnerability...[2]

This statement amounts to a condemnation of practices which sometimes take place in hospitals and in which nurses may be called on to participate. Given that a document such as a code of ethics, which has to be brief and to the point and cannot examine particular types of problem in any detail, can nevertheless issue uncompromising condemnations of this kind, we may come to ask ourselves: Is a properly-formulated code of professional conduct *sufficient* to enable a nurse to decide about the rightness or wrongness of alternative courses of action? Or do we need something more which no mere code, no matter how expertly drafted, could ever provide?

[1.] RCN code, p. 1.
[2.] RCN code, p. 2.

The answer is that we do need more, and that a code of professional conduct, by itself, can only state some basic principles governing right conduct, those principles needing to be interpreted, supplemented and developed in various ways. There are several reasons for this. First, even though some practices, such as harmful experimentation on patients, are so obviously contrary to the whole ethos of nursing that they can be condemned unequivocally in a code of ethics, a nurse may experience considerable difficulty in deciding whether a particular treatment in which she is asked to participate really does come under this heading or not: is it "a measure which jeopardises the safety of patients"?; does it amount to an "unnecessary treatment" or a "hazardous experimental procedure"? The correct application of these terms is not always easy and often requires careful thought. This is true also of very general prescriptions such as "The nurse, in providing care, promotes an environment in which the values, customs and spiritual beliefs of the individual are respected."[1] How does one decide that in a particular case a person's values, customs and spiritual beliefs are *not* being respected? The codes themselves give us no help in reaching such a conclusion; for this purpose we need, not only to reflect more carefully about what is being done to the patient, but also to examine certain basic questions concerning morality, such as: What does "failure to respect an individual's values, customs and spiritual beliefs" really amount to? And why is it wrong to show this lack of respect? These questions are far too basic to be resoluble in the brief compass of a code of nursing ethics. Such codes are inevitably stated in general terms which require much filling-out if their provisions are to be applied in concrete situations; and this filling-out is by no means a straightforward, quasi-mechanical process but requires careful reflexion on the facts of the case and on fundamental issues of morality.

A second drawback of codes of professional conduct arises from the fact that nurses often disagree among themselves about the morality of co-operation in various practices – in non-treatment of severely-handicapped neonates, for instance, or in sterilization procedures or programmes of *in vitro* fertilization. Because of this, we can expect that most codes will be drafted in such a way as to accommodate conflicting points of view. That is, those who draft the codes, recognizing that nurses disagree sharply over certain moral problems, will deliberately phrase

---

[1] ICN code, p. 2.

what they say so as not to favour one side or another in these controversies. But many of the perplexing difficulties which arise in nursing are, as one would expect, precisely problems on which people's viewpoints conflict: problems concerned with abortion and euthanasia, with contraception and sterilization and other issues in sexual ethics, with telling lies to patients and so on. One can hardly look for guidance concerning these matters to codes of ethics which have been deliberately phrased in order to leave each of them an open question! Of course, codes issued by nursing bodies which are committed to more detailed moral positions will offer far more specific guidance than those which deliberately skate over controverted matters. For instance, the 1986 CICIAMS code states that "Nurses cannot condone, nor co-operate directly in, any act that is contrary to the moral law. An act that deliberately destroys human life, or aims directly at decreasing or destroying the physical or psychological integrity of the person is always wrong". This provision is taken to apply to those human beings who have not yet attained effectively the "ability to exercise [their] responsibility as man..."[1] Since this statement evidently excludes abortion, it would be rejected by those nurses who believe abortion to be sometimes justified. We have to ask, then: "Is this assertion in the CICIAMS code justified, and if so why?" – a question which we can answer only by going back behind the codes themselves to the fundamental moral issues which have to be resolved *before* a concrete moral problem is tackled. Likewise, the RCN code, as we have seen, rules out striking as a means of pursuing legitimate industrial aims in nursing. ("Measures which jeopardise the safety of patients, such as ... the withdrawal of professional services during employment disputes, should be actively opposed by the profession as a whole.") But some other codes deliver no blanket condemnation of striking, and some explicitly allow it.[2] Where does the truth lie here? To decide this we are obliged, once again, to go beyond the professional codes and do some critical thinking for ourselves.

A third point is that those who draw up codes of ethics are by no means infallible, and that when they state some overall principle or approve or

---

[1] CICIAMS, *Code of Ethics* (Rome, 1986), paras. 3.2 and 3.3.

[2] See, e.g., the CICIAMS code, paragraph 2.4b: "The *right to strike*, which is a fundamental right of workers, applies to health personnel. It must have the purpose of defending legitimate professional interests as well as the guarantee of conditions which maintain the quality of care. However, problems arise which may prove difficult to resolve, with the result that irreparable damage to the sick is caused. Thus, essential care must always be safeguarded."

condemn some particular practice, they could be mistaken. Consider, for instance, the following statement of fundamental principles in the RCN code:

> The primary responsibility of nurses is to protect and enhance the wellbeing and dignity of each individual person in their care... Therefore it follows that:

> 1. Nursing care should be directed towards the preservation, or restoration as far as is possible, of a person's ability to function normally and independently within his own chosen environment.

And a gloss on this provision speaks of

> ... the *primary* end of nursing, which is to enable people to live their own lives as fully and freely as possible by providing professional counsel and care according to particular needs.[1]

Many readers of the RCN code would probably accept these statements as clearly true, and certainly the duties ascribed to the nurse in this passage really are duties for her: she is obliged to protect and enhance her patients' well-being and dignity, to enable them to live full and free lives, and so on. But on reflexion we can see that some of the statements quoted above are at least disputable. Only on the basis of an all-encompassing definition of health like that of the World Health Organization could this conception of the primary end of nursing be defended; and, as we have seen, such an all-encompassing definition of health is open to objection. It seems more reasonable to say that the primary end of nursing is the promotion of the health or bodily well-being of the patient, but that since the patient is not just a living body but a *person*, nurses must treat him in ways which respect his personal nature, of which his bodily nature is only one aspect. The question at issue is, of course, one of emphasis and priorities; but it is arguable that the RCN code has its priorities wrong in this passage. So, in general, although we should expect cases of actual error in codes of ethics to be rare, we should never regard the codes as sacrosanct.

This awkward fact of the fallibility of all professional codes would remain even if the first two objections to an uncritical reliance on them could somehow be overcome. Suppose that we had a code of professional conduct which was sufficiently voluminous to cover a wide range of

---

[1.] RCN code, p. 1.

ethical problems and which faced all the major ethical issues squarely, without skating over any of them because of disagreements among nurses themselves. It would remain the case that this code, precisely because it had been composed by fallible human beings, would itself be fallible. Recently, a draft code on confidentiality was issued by the Department of Health and Social Security. Because this code focused specifically on one aspect of health-care ethics, that of confidentiality, it could be seen as an attempt to supplement the very rudimentary guidance provided by the codes of professional conduct and thus to make up for their necessary brevity. But this draft code on confidentiality came in for fierce criticism from the UKCC and other nursing organizations on the grounds that it would enable health professionals to disclose confidential information about patients far too easily and would therefore threaten the rights of patients.[1] So there is nothing "untouchable" about codes of professional conduct: they are no more immune from criticism than any other statement or document composed by fallible human beings.

One final word against the idea that codes of professional conduct give nurses all that they need for deciding how to act in difficult situations. The codes which we have looked at all place great emphasis on working for the genuine good of the patient as the primary goal of all the nurse's activities. As the UKCC code puts it, the nurse must "act always in such a way as to promote and safeguard the well-being and interests of patients/clients."[2] Now if one is to act on this injunction, one must first of all be clear about just what kinds of change in the patient's condition would be genuinely beneficial to him and what others would not. Suppose that the problem is whether or not to resuscitate an elderly patient suffering cardiac arrest. Following the code's advice, we ask: "Would it be in the patient's *interest* to be resuscitated? Would we be *doing him good* if we were to resuscitate him?"; and only if we can answer "Yes" should we go ahead and resuscitate. The codes of professional conduct, however, provide us with no resources for answering these questions. In order, therefore, to apply the principle that concern for the patient's good is crucial, one must first grasp what sorts of things *are* for the patient's good and what are not.

This point is important because health professionals sometimes attempt to justify treatment or non-treatment of patients by reference to

---

[1] Cf. article "UKCC upset at new confidentiality code", *Nursing Times*, vol. 83, no. 32 (August 12–18, 1987), p. 6.
[2] UKCC code, p. 2.

the patient's good when in fact their decisions are based on morally dubious "quality-of-life" considerations. If, for instance, a doctor says "This patient should not be resuscitated because that wouldn't really benefit him" (or: ". . . because that wouldn't do him any good"), he may be expressing a quality-of-life criterion for deciding on treatment or non-treatment. He would then be saying that if someone is unable to perform reasonably well certain characteristically human activities, such as thinking coherently, talking with other people, and so on, his life is not of a sufficiently high quality to justify health professionals in intervening to keep it going. Paediatricians who refuse to treat handicapped newborn infants who are capable of benefiting from treatment – babies with severe spina bifida and some degree of mental impairment, for instance – often take this same attitude. They would say also that it is not in their patients' own interests to be kept alive; the infants should rather be helped to die by having all life-preserving treatment and care (including adequate nutrition) withheld from them. This kind of attitude is in many ways suspect, not least because the dubious claims which are made about quality of life and "worthwhileness" and "the patient's interest" are evidently untestable. When a consultant says that adequate nutrition for a child is ruled out because it is not in his own interest, how can he be sure that this is the case? How does he work out what is in the patient's interest and what is not? May he not be motivated by a purely private feeling about the matter, or, even worse, by a positive desire to rid the world of certain types of patients whom he regards as "better off dead"? At any rate, whatever answer we give to these questions, the codes of professional conduct cannot help us. For these codes all tend to employ the notion of the patient's interest without giving us criteria for applying this notion in particular cases. If we do decide that some treatment or other is or is not in the patient's interest, we shall already have to have decided on the criteria for judging one way or the other; and this involves our going well beyond the codes of professional conduct to concentrate on basic concepts and arguments of ethics as applied to nursing practice. There is no way of avoiding a consideration of these basic ethical concepts and arguments, and the sooner we settle down to the business of examining them the better. They will be the focus of discussion in the next few chapters.

★ ★ ★

This Chapter in Summary

Codes of professional conduct play an important role in modern nursing practice in setting out basic standards of practice to which nurses are expected to adhere. A careful look at some codes reveals that they corroborate the account of nursing and the nurse's role set out in Chapter One. While codes of professional conduct are useful documents as expressing concisely the basic attitudes and standards to which the nursing profession is committed, we would be wrong to place too high a value on them. A nurse needs much more than a knowledge of codes of ethics if she is to deal intelligently with ethical problems; in particular, she must be able to "get behind" the codes, to appreciate the spirit which they express, and to think critically and independently about the important moral issues.

CHAPTER THREE

PHILOSOPHY, ETHICS AND NURSING ETHICS

Many of the moral problems which arise in nursing practice are complex and highly perplexing. If we are to deal adequately with these problems we shall first have to pose some general, and quite fundamental, questions concerning morality itself – what morality is, how it comes about that some things are right or wrong, and so on. More precisely, we must pay some attention to such questions as the following:

What does it mean to say that some action is good or bad, right or wrong? And how do we know that any action is good or bad, right or wrong?

What connexion is there between morality and human happiness? Should we regard acts as good or right if they tend to promote happiness?

What do we mean by people's *rights* to do certain things or to receive certain benefits? Can we resolve important moral disputes by appealing to people's possession of rights?

Are there any actions which in themselves, and regardless of their consequences, are evil and therefore not to be engaged in? If so, what are these actions?

All these questions have a kind of ultimacy and a degree of abstractness which make them essentially *philosophical* questions. That is, they are questions which are traditionally part of the study of philosophy and which require, for their proper handling, a type of reflective thinking which is philosophical in character. In the next few chapters we shall, then, raise some typical questions of moral philosophy, only afterwards returning to consider in detail the various difficulties arising from nursing practice.

Philosophical issues are typically not resoluble (as are problems in mathematics, for example) by the straightforward application of a standard procedure yielding a definite and generally accepted solution. On the contrary, there is no consensus among philosophers as to the solution of central philosophical problems. In fact, probably all the issues which were hotly disputed by Socrates, Plato, Aristotle and others in ancient Athens are still live issues today, on which philosophers hold conflicting views. Hence the discussion of moral arguments and basic moral principles in this and the next two chapters cannot pretend to provide anything like a comprehensive treatment of the subject. Certainly it will expound the basic "moves" which appear to be required for resolving the issues · treated, but it would be over-ambitious to aim for much more than this.

The major part of this chapter, then, will be concerned with the nature of philosophy and philosophical argument, and in particular with philosophical argument as applied to issues of moral good and evil, right and wrong; and at the end of the chapter I shall also say something about nursing ethics as a kind of "applied ethics" in which general moral principles are applied to problems arising in nursing practice.

Philosophy and religious belief: an objection

Do we really need to immerse ourselves in all these philosophical issues? Is there not a more direct way of approaching the crucial problems of nursing ethics? The suggestion that there is such a short-cut might be made on religious grounds. For a committed Christian might urge that instead of trying to guide ourselves by our own notoriously fallible powers of reasoning, we should take our stand on God's revelation, where we are far more likely to receive genuine enlightenment. We should act on St. Paul's injunction to "search the scriptures" in pursuit of the assistance and moral guidance which we need. Is this suggestion a reasonable one? Well, we should not dismiss it out of hand, because much of what is said in scripture does have important implications for medical and nursing ethics. There is, for example, the uncompromising condemnation of killing the innocent in the Book of Exodus,[1] and the various texts which appear to accept human foetuses as actual human beings, not merely potential ones.[2] Texts such as these are clearly relevant to debates over issues such as euthanasia and abortion. However, it is unlikely that

---

[1]   "Do not bring death on an innocent man that has justice on his side" (Exodus 23, 7). (All biblical quotations are from the Knox translation, unless otherwise stated.)

[2]   See, e.g., Jeremiah 1, 4–6: "The word of the Lord came to me, and his message was: I claimed thee for my own before ever I fashioned thee in thy mother's womb; before ever thou camest to the birth, I set thee apart for myself."

an *exclusive* reliance on scriptural texts would get us very far, because what we are given in the scriptures is not sufficiently detailed to handle the sheer complexity of moral problems in medicine and nursing. Hence we need to view the scriptural texts themselves in the light of what one can discover about fundamental ethical principles by using one's natural reasoning; and to do this is, of course, to give up any exclusive reliance on the scriptures and engage in philosophical thinking as well. To see this, let us consider more closely the two passages just referred to. First, the text condemning the killing of the innocent. Suppose we want to determine whether or not this condemnation applies to some particular human act which results in someone's death. For this purpose we may need to ask a number of questions which the Bible itself gives us few resources for answering, such as: (1) Is this condemnation of killing the innocent meant to apply to all such killings, or does it apply only generally and for the most part? If the latter, there could be extreme circumstances in which the consequences of *not* killing the innocent would be so appalling that we could rightly make an exception to the general rule. (2) Who exactly counts as "innocent", anyway? What about a civilian population who, in wartime, enthusiastically support their government's war effort and try to assist their fighting men by working intensely hard at their jobs? Are they to be considered as innocent and therefore as immune from direct military attack by the other side, or as combatants and therefore as legitimate targets? Secondly, consider the other biblical text, in which the human foetus is apparently recognized as a full human being. How far does this notion extend? It would certainly apply to any unborn child who was fairly close to being born, but one might doubt whether one which was less well-developed, such as an eight-week-old foetus, would be similarly covered. And what about a one-day-old embryo, which, to judge solely by appearances, has nothing in common with a fully-developed member of the human species? These questions are evidently unanswerable as long as our only resource for answering them is what we find in the Bible itself.

We cannot, then, seize on such isolated scriptural texts, extremely valuable though they are, as an excuse for not doing any hard mental work ourselves. On the contrary, if we are to understand the biblical texts correctly and grasp their bearing on many ethical problems, we must first have reached some convictions about what it is for something to be right or wrong. It is the aim of the philosopher to investigate these questions in a rigorous way and to propose answers to them.

Philosophy and Catholic moral teaching

Bioethical problems cannot, then, be solved by a mere reliance on the scriptures as the word of God. However, this is not quite the end of the argument on this score. For suppose that our opponent of philosophy is not just "a committed Christian", as he was initially described, but a Catholic. Then he can claim that although the Bible itself is not sufficient for our task, since it has to be interpreted and filled out in various ways, the Catholic believer can appeal to an accredited and authoritative interpreter of the sacred text, the Church's living *magisterium*. So a Catholic would regard an official Vatican statement on bioethical issues such as the one issued on euthanasia in 1980, authorized by the Pope himself, as giving authoritative guidance on disputed bioethical matters in the light of the faith.[1]

However, it is hard to believe that a simple acceptance of the Church's authoritative teaching could ever be sufficient for a Catholic who is attempting to resolve problems in nursing ethics. There are at least three reasons for thinking that something more is required.

First, although the Catholic's acceptance of the Church's *magisterium* as an authoritative interpreter of the Bible and expositor of the Catholic faith enables *him* to hold with certitude definite conclusions on controverted moral issues, he can hardly expect this commitment of his to cut any ice with those who do not share his faith. He cannot, for example, reasonably expect a non-Catholic to reject a certain practice (*in vitro* fertilization, for example) just because it is condemned in a papal encyclical. So if his only ground for holding to his moral convictions is that these convictions are in accord with the mind of the Church, he can have little of interest to say to people of other religions or no religion at all. But this is a severe drawback, surely: the Catholic *should* be able to contribute something to the thoughts of the conscientious non-Catholic who is trying to decide how he should approach crucial issues of right and wrong; he should not be incapable of making any contact with the non-Catholic's outlook.

Secondly, if God forbids some practice, it can normally be assumed that the practice is in itself wrong, and that He forbids it precisely because it is wrong. Likewise, if God commands that we engage in a certain

---

[1] Sacred Congregation for the Doctrine of the Faith, *Declaration on Euthanasia* (Vatican City, 1980).

practice – in regular prayer, for example – we can assume that He enjoins the practice on us because it is an intrinsically good one. In other words, God does not command us to do X or forbid us to do Y for no reason at all. As a rule, then, God forbids things because they are wrong in themselves; we cannot normally suppose that they are wrong solely because He forbids them. (It may sometimes be the case that God enjoins some practice on us not because that practice is the only appropriate and morally right one, but simply because there must be some uniform practice among rational beings, and that practice is as good as any – just as it does not matter whether motorists drive on the right or the left, as long as they all drive on the same side of the road. But it is hardly likely that cases of this sort would be common: normally, if God enjoins some practice it is because the practice is good in itself, and if He forbids a practice it is because it is bad in itself.) But in this case, since men are rational creatures, "made in the image and likeness of God" by their possession of reason and free will, they should be able to understand, at least in part, *why* certain actions are right and certain other actions are wrong. Admittedly, human beings have finite intelligences; they cannot plumb the depths of the created universe and apprehend the *raison d'être* of everything that exists. But a certain limited understanding of why things are as they are is, at least, open to them. So in the moral sphere we should expect that human beings will be able to grasp, to some extent, the basic principles of morality and the way in which these principles should be applied. The Catholic Church itself teaches that people can in principle achieve a basic grasp of what is morally right and wrong without having to rely on God's revelation. This is largely the point of the doctrine of *the natural moral law* which Catholic moral philosophers and theologians have, over the years, investigated and tried to develop.

Thirdly, authoritative statements of the Church's *magisterium* often enunciate general principles without indicating how these principles should be applied in particular cases. If a nurse, say, is to utilize the general principles so as to work out what to do in this particular case, she will have to give up any simple reliance on magisterial documents and do some hard thinking for herself – a task which will be successful only if she understands the *point* of the general principles enunciated by the Church.

A Catholic is not, therefore, absolved by his faith in God and his acceptance of the Church's teachings from the obligation to think rationally about things – and this applies to thinking about bioethical issues just as much as anything else. To say this is not to rule out all appeals to God's revelation and Christian tradition in resolving crucial moral issues, but simply to reject a totally one-sided reliance on revealed teachings. The fact that man's intellectual powers are limited means that we may well have to rely, in various ways, on truths communicated to us through revelation and tradition, and some of these ways are indicated in later chapters. A Christian may well say that fundamental problems of morality will be adequately handled only if we make use of *both* independent philosophical reasoning and God's revelation as interpreted in Christian tradition.[1] But for the moment the philosophical side of this twofold picture needs to be emphasized, because philosophical reasoning is something with which many people are unfamiliar and which therefore needs to be described in some detail. In the next chapter I shall consider some philosophical questions concerning the nature of morality. But in this chapter I discuss three questions of a more elementary nature about philosophy in general, in the hope that this discussion will be of particular help to readers who have not previously studied philosophy. These questions are:

(1) What is philosophy, and how do we proceed when we are thinking about philosophical issues? And just what is a philosophical issue, anyway – how is it distinguished from other kinds of issue?

(2) What is ethics, and what are the crucial problems with which it deals? How do we proceed in dealing with difficult ethical problems?

(3) What is "nursing ethics", and how is it related to ethics in general?

These three questions will be considered, very briefly, in turn.

What is philosophy?

In one sense the question "What is philosophy?" is easily answered, in another it is not. We can reach the easy answer simply by listing the major

---

[1]   For a helpful exploration of some ways in which Christian faith can impinge on people's ethical beliefs, see G. G. Grisez, "Practical Reasoning and Christian Faith", *Proceedings of the American Catholic Philosophical Association*, vol. 58, 1984, pp. 2–14. G. J. Hughes, in his *Authority in Morals* (London, 1978), strongly criticizes the idea that Christian ethics can do without philosophy and be based solely on God's revelation.

types of issue with which philosophy deals, without explaining why it is appropriate that these issues should be dealt with by philosophy rather than some other subject, or what gives philosophical thinking the power to deal with them. So, for instance, one might propose the following definition. "Philosophy is the discipline which examines and attempts to resolve such questions as the following: the existence and nature of God; the nature of man (including the question whether man is a purely material being or a composite of matter and spirit); the existence of free will in man and other rational beings; the nature of rationality and the forms of argument in which it expresses itself; the nature of causality and of space and time; the meaning of moral words such as 'good', 'evil', 'right', 'wrong', 'duty', 'ought'; the criteria for deciding whether or not a proposed human action is morally right; the justification of political authority; and so on." Now while such an enumeration of topics would give us some understanding of what philosophy is about, it would leave us lamentably ignorant of its true nature. For the topics listed are not considered only by the philosopher: God is studied also in theology, the nature of man in psychology, space, time and causal interactions in physics, the meanings of words in lexicography, and so on. What, then, is so special about the philosopher's examination of these subjects? How does it differ from that of the others? Evidently, defining philosophy simply by listing some typical philosophical problems would do nothing to enlighten us on any of these points. We need, then, to leave behind this purely "external" characterization of philosophy in terms of the range of topics dealt with, and instead come to grips with it "from the inside", so to speak, by examining the way in which the philosopher tries to solve particular problems, and the features of his subject matter upon which he fastens his attention. When we take this approach, however, the question "What is philosophy?" is no longer easy but extremely difficult to answer. In fact, this question is itself a philosophical question, about which different practitioners of the subject hold different and often conflicting views. Since no purely "external" view of philosophy can succeed in conveying its nature adequately, the best way of grasping what philosophy amounts to is to get to grips with some actual philosophical problems. This is what will be attempted in the next few chapters. For the moment, the following summary remarks are intended only to give some overall impressions of philosophy which the investigations of the next few chapters will, it is hoped, fill out.

One way in which philosophy differs from other disciplines is the fact that many philosophical questions have a fundamentally general and abstract character. As one writer puts it:

> ... philosophy distinguishes itself from the other sciences by its point of view. For when it takes an object into consideration, it sees it exclusively from the standpoint, so to speak, of the borderline, of the fundamental aspects. In this sense, philosophy is a science of foundations. At the point where other sciences come to a standstill, where they assume conditions without further investigation, that is where the philosopher first begins to question. The other sciences attain knowledge – he asks what knowledge is; the other sciences establish laws – he asks what a law is. The average man and the politician speak about meaning and purpose, but the philosopher asks what actually should be understood by meaning and purpose. Thus, philosophy is a radical science in the sense that it gets closer to the roots of the matter than the other sciences, and that it wants to question and investigate further at that point where the others are satisfied.[1]

It is not surprising, then, that philosophical questions typically take a form such as "What is X?" (where "X" stands for an abstract noun such as "time" or "beauty" or "goodness") or "What is it for X to be Y?" (as, for example, "What is it for one event to be the cause of another?"; "What is it for a word to have a meaning?"; "What is it for something to exist?"). Not all philosophical questions have this abstract, general character – the question "Does God exist?", for example, does not, since it is concerned with the being or non-being of an individual entity rather than with the nature of some kind of thing or characteristic – but many of them are of this sort. *All* philosophical questions, however, are questions which cannot be solved either by human reasoning functioning at the level of common sense, as in one's dealings with everyday domestic or business transactions, or by the physical or social sciences. In this sense philosophical thinking takes us beyond both common-sense thought and the sciences. The fact that physical science is incapable of solving philosophical problems should be emphasized, because many people today seem to be obsessed with the idea that science is omnicompetent. The fact is that

---

[1] J. M. Bochenski, *Philosophy: An Introduction* (New York, 1972), p. 28.

although one needs to know about the relevant findings of modern science if one is to handle many philosophical problems intelligently, such problems can never be solved merely by applying to them techniques developed in (say) physics or biology.

Why is this? Well, philosophy goes beyond the conclusions of the experimental sciences in three ways. First, the results established by the sciences themselves raise questions which the experimental method employed by scientists is powerless to solve. So, for instance, there are difficulties in understanding how the conclusions reached in relativity theory or quantum physics are to be "squared" with our ordinary, common-sense ways of understanding the world. Can the scientific and the common-sense approaches be combined harmoniously, or do we have to write off one of them as giving us a false picture of reality? Plenty of scientists have tried to clarify this sort of issue, but in doing so they have been speaking not as scientists but rather as philosophers of science, since there is no way of resolving these problems without going beyond the experimental method which is the scientific researcher's constant tool.

The second way in which philosophical speculation goes beyond science is by trying to justify the fundamental beliefs which scientists presuppose in their work. Thus, science could not get off the ground unless the scientist assumed that the universe is orderly in the sense that the laws governing the behaviour of things, whatever these laws might be, hold not just at certain times and in certain places, but always and everywhere. Suppose that scientists did not make this assumption but believed instead that a scientific law – the law of universal gravitation, for instance – might at any time cease to hold, or that it might sometimes hold in one place but not in another. If this were admitted as a real possibility, the scientist could not confidently draw any conclusions from the results of his experiments. If, then, he is to reach any definite conclusions at all, he must assume that the universe is orderly and that the basic laws of nature are constant and invariable. But since this assumption of order in the universe is presupposed in all scientific work it cannot itself be explained or accounted for by scientific means. On the other hand, some explanation for the orderliness of the universe is needed, because on the face of it there is no reason why the universe should be orderly rather than chaotic, that is, why physical entities should behave in accordance with constant and unchanging laws, rather than no laws at all, or laws which change suddenly and capriciously from one moment to the next. At the very least, we can easily *imagine* a thoroughly chaotic universe, and there seems no obvious intrinsic impossibility in there being such a universe. So why is our universe orderly rather than chaotic? If we are to answer this question we shall have to go beyond all the established conclusions of science and proceed by what we might call "pure philosophical reasoning". It might be urged that this question is in fact insoluble, that we can never come to know why the universe is orderly but must accept it as a brute fact. But this conclusion would have to be *argued for*, and any such argument would again be a philosophical argument.[1]

Again, the scientist bases his experimental work on his understanding of certain fundamental laws of nature which past scientific research has established, such as the law of universal gravitation or the statistical laws of quantum physics. He presupposes the truth of these laws of nature in all his work, but *as a scientist* he does not ask what it is for these laws to hold – whether, for example, the fact that these laws do hold is a mere matter of fact about the universe, or whether, on the other hand, there is some fundamental reason in the nature of things why physical bodies should behave in the way specified by the law, and if so what this fundamental reason is. Likewise the scientist, along with the man of common sense, takes for granted the existence of physical substances and endeavours to explain the way in which these physical substances behave, how they combine with each other to form chemical compounds, how they exert pressure on other bodies, and so on. A physicist may concern himself with the problem of how the universe came into being from more primitive states of matter, but he does not ask why the objects which we observe through our senses actually exist rather than not. But the philosopher – or more precisely the metaphysician, since this question arises in the most fundamental "part" of philosophy, metaphysics – may go beyond the problems posed by the scientist, and ask: "Why should this particular being (this dog Fido, this fountain pen in my pocket, I myself) exist at this very moment?" For he sees that there is nothing in the nature of all these things that necessitates their existence, and that the mere fact that they were brought into being at some previous point in time and

---

[1]. The kind of questioning illustrated here, concerning the orderliness of the universe, provides the basis for one of the traditional arguments for God's existence, the so-called teleological argument, or argument from order or design. See B. Davies, *Thinking about God* (London, 1985), pp. 35–60, and R. Swinburne, *The Existence of God* (Oxford, 1980), pp. 133–157.

through such-and-such a process does nothing to explain their existence here and now. He recognizes, that is, that the present existence of all these things needs to be explained, and that the explanation will have to be of a different kind from that which is standard in physical science. It is on the basis of such considerations that one of the most important philosophical arguments for the existence of God – known generally as the contingency argument, or the argument from the contingency of the world – has been built up.[1]

A third way in which philosophy goes beyond the results established by the sciences is by examining and trying to solve problems which, as far as we can tell, have no obvious relation to scientific theories and conclusions, so that the various sciences are largely irrelevant to their resolution. Questions in aesthetics (most fundamentally, perhaps, the question "What is beauty?") and in ethics are of this sort. How, for instance, could one bring the resources of modern physics or biochemistry to bear upon such a question as "What is it for a human action to be right or wrong?" It would be rash to say that scientific results are totally irrelevant to the task of answering these questions, but the connexion between the two – the philosophical questions and the scientific results – is at best tenuous.

Philosophical problems appear, then, to be ultimate in the sense that it is beyond the resources of any of the special sciences to answer them. They cannot, that is, be resolved by the method characteristic of physical science, which is that of testing hypotheses by suitably-designed experiments. Philosophy should also be clearly distinguished from theology. For the philosopher proceeds by relying solely on his natural power of reasoning, without appealing to divine revelation. He may well be a convinced Christian, believing, on the authority of God's word, in such fundamental Christian doctrines as those concerning the Trinity, the divinity of Christ and His incarnation, crucifixion and resurrection, the Church as the Mystical Body of Christ and so on. But *as a philosopher* he attempts to establish his conclusions solely on the basis of considerations which are knowable by the natural light of reason, prescinding from the truths which divine revelation has taught him. He may, of course, be influenced and guided in all sorts of ways by his religious beliefs; but the *arguments* which he produces for his conclusions, if they are to be

---

[1]. For an exposition of the contingency argument, see E. L. Mascall, *He Who Is* (London: 1943), pp. 40–82; B. Davies, *Thinking about God*, pp. 17–32 ; G. G. Grisez, *Beyond the New Theism* (Notre Dame, 1974), pp. 36–91.

philosophical arguments rather than theological ones, will make no appeal to religious beliefs or presuppositions, but will be based on conclusions available in principle to men of all religious beliefs and none.

An illustration: questioning the foundations of morality

A fresh example, this time about morality, will help to illustrate the distinction between common-sense and philosophical thinking. A man who is trying to decide whether he should change his will in such a way as to benefit one of his children more than the others asks himself: "Would it be right for me to do this? Do I not have a duty to maintain the present clauses of the will favouring all the children equally? Or am I entitled to go ahead with this proposed change?" Now these questions are not, of course, philosophical questions; they are practical moral questions about what the man ought to do. Suppose, however, that as a result of his agonizing over these practical problems, he begins to ask more general questions such as the following: "Just what does it mean, anyway, to say that some action is right or wrong, or that it is my duty to do it? Then again, how do I know that something is right or wrong or my duty – in other words, what are the criteria for making such a judgment? And what makes those criteria correct? Is it, in fact, really the case that some actions are good and some evil in themselves and regardless of the attitudes which people take towards them? Or is it that nothing is really good or bad in itself, but that we all have an irresistible tendency to think in this way?" All these questions, which any reflective person may easily find himself asking, are philosophical questions; they are of a different order from those which originally worried our hesitant testator, because they deal, not with the rights and wrongs of a particular kind of action, but with right and wrong as such, with what makes something to be right or wrong, and with how we can recognize something to be right or wrong. The fact that people can easily be led from a consideration of concrete moral questions to pose abstract philosophical issues of this type does not mean that they are usually well-equipped to resolve them. Far from it: unless they have already developed an aptitude for disciplined philosophical thinking, the likelihood is that they will regard these issues as hopelessly difficult and abandon any attempt to think them through. Perhaps, indeed, they will come to doubt whether such questions really have any answers, or, even if they do, whether any human being could ever find the answers.

The question of philosophical method

If people do react in this way, by writing off philosophical issues as insoluble, this may be because there is no obvious way of handling them; for philosophical problems cannot be resolved by appealing to divine revelation, or by observing what is going on in the world, or by conducting scientific experiments. For this reason someone who was sceptical about the value of philosophy might issue the following challenge: "If, by philosophizing, one can acquire knowledge of things which is not obtainable either from scientific research or from observation of the world, this must be because the philosopher has a special method of inquiry which enables him to derive conclusions which are unobtainable without it. What, then, is this method? It is up to the philosopher to describe it, and to defend its adequacy as a means of reaching the truth, if his claims on behalf of philosophy are to be taken seriously."

This question is a difficult one to answer, because on the face of it there is no single method of thinking and arguing which is employed by philosophers but rather a host of such methods. Hence, as one writer has said, we cannot "define precisely what the method of philosophy is except at the expense of grotesquely limiting the subject". For, he goes on:

> Philosophy has not just one method but a variety of different methods according to its subject-matter, and no useful purpose is served by defining them in advance of their application... Philosophy requires a great variety of methods, for it must draw into its service and subject to its interpretation all kinds of human experience... [The philosopher] must aim at giving a systematic consistent picture of human experience and of the world in which as much is explained as can from the nature of the case admit of explanation...[1]

Talk of "*the* method employed in philosophy" is, then, likely to be misleading, since the philosopher will proceed in different ways according to the kind of problem which he is treating.[2] It is, indeed, arguable that there is no one method of investigation which is proper to the

---

[1] A. C. Ewing, *The Fundamental Questions of Philosophy* (London, 1952), pp. 20–21.
[2] J. M. Bochenski's work *The Methods of Contemporary Thought* (Dordrecht, 1965) is a useful short account of some of the methods followed by contemporary philosophers.

philosopher in the sense that it is used *only* in philosophical speculation and argument. What sets philosophy apart from other fields of study is that the philosopher calls our attention to certain features of our daily lives that we are all inclined to ignore, especially if we are preoccupied with everyday business or family concerns. He points out, for instance, certain features of the way we use words such as "right" and "wrong", thereby indicating certain aspects of the *reality* which we describe by those words. Or the philosopher may point out certain features of *finitude* and *limitation* in the things around us, or in human beings themselves, and go on from there to argue that the existence of beings with this finite or limited character can be accounted for only if we accept that there exists a being who is not subject to any sort of limitation. (This pattern of argument is exemplified in most of the traditional arguments for the existence of God.) Or he may fasten his gaze upon certain important features of our inner mental lives and argue that such features could not in principle be displayed by any purely physical or material being, and hence that there is in man some "element" or "component" which is appropriately called "a spiritual soul". In all these examples of philosophical reasoning what we have is not any one type or pattern of argument which is exclusively philosophical. Rather, there is a use of types of argument which are to be met with also in science and common-sense reasoning, but based on a kind of observation or scrutiny which seizes on features of things normally taken for granted in day-to-day life.[1] It is, then, the *use* which the philosopher makes of the various methods of thought which is characteristic of philosophical procedure, not the methods of thought considered just in themselves.

Ethics and Nursing Ethics

Since philosophy is all about seeking fundamental explanations for the fact that the things in the world exist and are what they are, it is clear that philosophy is divisible into a number of separate subjects according to the type of thing or being on which attention is focussed. One very general body of philosophical reasoning will centre on the question: "What is it for a thing – anything at all, of whatever kind – simply *to be*, to be *a*

[1.] A much fuller account of this attitude towards philosophy will be found in F. C. Copleston's article "Philosophical Knowledge" (in H. D. Lewis, ed., *Contemporary British Philosophy*, Third Series (London, 1956), pp. 119–140).

being?", and this highly general, abstract and fundamental part of philosophy is called metaphysics. Then, according as we concentrate more narrowly on particular kinds of things – on physical substances and their activities, on human beings, on activities such as scientific investigation and aesthetic appreciation – we shall have such disciplines as, respectively, philosophy of nature, philosophy of man, philosophy of science and aesthetics. That branch of philosophy which is called ethics or moral philosophy involves investigating the data of morality. It seeks, first of all, to discover whether what we might call "the facts of morality" (e.g., that murder is wrong, that one should not act against one's conscience) really are facts, and secondly, to identify the fundamental reasons why these facts (provided we find them to be such) are as they are. So ethics focuses on such notions as those of good and bad, right and wrong, duty, obligation, etc., and on such questions as: "Are our moral judgments capable of being justified? If so, how?", "What does it mean to say that someone is responsible for his actions?", "What is the point of praising and blaming people for their conduct?", "How can the practice of punishing those whom we call 'evildoers' be justified?", and so on.

Here we have a whole range of difficult and contentious issues, all of them calling for the philosopher's careful attention. But there is one ethical question which appears to be more important than all the others, because the way in which we answer it will do much to determine our approach to those others, and to practical moral difficulties. This central question is: Are there objective facts concerning morality? Is it a fact that certain things are good and certain others bad, or that certain human acts are right and certain others wrong? Suppose, for example, that somebody asserts that destructive experimentation on human subjects is wrong. Is he saying something either true or false about the practice of human experimentation, just as a man who said "I am now sitting at a desk, writing a letter to my wife" would be saying something true or false? If what he says is true, we can conclude that the wrongness or otherwise of human experimentation is somehow a real or objective feature of that practice, and that in general we are capable of rationally apprehending certain facts about the states of affairs and actions which we evaluate morally. But if this is not so then we cannot regard our moral judgments as informing us about the way things are. On this view, moral knowledge either does not exist or is a matter entirely of people's personal tastes and predilections, likes and dislikes, to which nothing in the nature of things corresponds. Either of these views, surely, would amount to an abandonment of morality as people normally understand it. Many people today do defend one or the other of these attitudes, but in the next chapter I shall argue that they are mistaken.

So much for ethics in general. How should we characterize nursing ethics in particular? Nursing ethics is the application of principles and patterns of argument employed in ethics to moral problems which typically arise in the course of a nurse's work. That is, we have, on the one hand, certain conclusions and also certain techniques of argumentation which are yielded by our study of general ethics; and on the other hand there are all the various kinds of ethical problem which present themselves for nurses in hospitals and health clinics, in doctors' surgeries, on health-visiting rounds, and so on. We attempt to resolve these problems of nursing practice by applying to them the conclusions and techniques yielded by a study of ethics in general. Nursing ethics is, then, one type of "applied ethics", along with medical ethics, business ethics, military ethics and so on. Now since nursing ethics does involve applying principles which come from a prior study of ethics in general, there can be no question of making valuable progress in nursing ethics unless one has sorted out some crucial issues in general ethics. This procedure will, then, be followed in the chapters to come: first, some very basic questions in ethics will be discussed, and then the conclusions drawn from this discussion will be applied to problems raised by nursing practice.

★ ★ ★

This Chapter in Summary

While our concern in this book is to tackle some of the pressing problems encountered by nurses in hospital wards and on health-visiting rounds, etc., we should be unwise to try to resolve these problems without further ado. For we cannot hope to resolve them without a good deal of prior argument, especially about certain more general issues which belong to ethics or moral philosophy. (It might be thought that we could avoid all involvement in philosophical issues by relying on God's revelation, either as given to us just in the Bible or as interpreted by the *magisterium* of the Catholic Church. But this will not do: even if there is an important place for appeals to God's revelation in bioethics, there are also questions which we can deal with only by arguing philosophically.) Since moral philosophy is a particular "part" or department of philosophy, we have to consider at some length what philosophy is and how philosophical enquiries differ from those carried out in other fields, particularly everyday practical enquiries and scientific research. Whereas general ethics is a particular "part" of philosophy, nursing ethics is a type of *applied* ethics, in which the principles and argumentative techniques built up in general ethics are applied to the particular problems raised by nursing practice.

CHAPTER FOUR

MORALITY AND OBJECTIVE TRUTH

In this and the following two chapters we shall be trying to tackle the question: Are there objective truths of morality? Is it the case that certain actions are good or bad, right or wrong *in themselves* and quite apart from what people happen to think about them? Would, for instance, the deliberate killing of an innocent person be immoral in itself, even if everyone who knew about the killing thoroughly approved of it? If the answer to all these questions is "Yes", it will follow that our moral judgments have two crucially important features. First, they are capable of being true or false, in a straightforward sense of these words. Secondly, if a moral judgment is true, this will be because of the nature of the act which the judgment is about, not because of anyone's personal attitude, either favourable or unfavourable, towards that act. I shall lump these two features together under the heading of "objectivity" and say that the aim of this and the following chapters is to decide whether the *objectivity* of moral beliefs and judgments can be rationally defended.

The problem of moral pluralism

It might be thought that the objectivity of morality, in this sense, is so obviously true that any attempt to establish it would be an unnecessary labour. After all, anyone who defends any moral viewpoint – that euthanasia is immoral, for example, or that we should support the less well-off members of society from our taxes – necessarily holds that his convictions are objectively true. He believes, that is, that there *are* truths of morality, truths which hold regardless of whether or not anybody ever recognizes them as such. And surely there are no reasonable grounds for doubting this? Why should anyone ever want to think otherwise?

The fact is, however, that many people – and not just academic philosophers – do apparently deny that someone who says "Hanging is a just punishment for those who commit cold-blooded murders" or "Lying is always wrong" is stating something which may be true or false. We have all, probably, come across people who hold that "What you believe about moral matters is really up to you", or that "You have to choose for yourself what your values are going to be". What these people seem to be saying is that moral problems are not problems to which there is ever a definitely right or a definitely wrong answer: one has to decide for oneself what moral outlook one should adopt towards capital punishment or euthanasia, etc., and this amounts to making a basic option which is not justifiable on any rational grounds and cannot be intelligibly regarded as objectively true or false. Consider the following exchange, in which the contribution of the second speaker, Peter, is typical of many actual ethical disagreements:

Jane: "I believe that lying to patients about their condition and prospects is always wrong."

Peter: "That just means that lying is wrong *to you*; but it may not be wrong to other people."

This remark, "It's wrong *to you*", is used to imply that what Jane has said merely expresses a subjective personal attitude towards lying which is devoid of any objective truth or falsity. Jane, on the other hand, had clearly meant to assert that lying was wrong as a matter of objective fact; so Peter's rejoinder amounts to a rejection of her assumption that there is truth and falsity in moral judgments. Hence the idea that there is no objective truth or falsity in morality is encountered frequently in everyday life. Why should this be the case?

The answer is that people's moral beliefs have certain features which are deeply puzzling, and which therefore provoke severe difficulties if we interpret those beliefs as describing the way things are. In particular, people's moral disagreements are often intractable in a way that other sorts of everyday disagreement are not. When two people disagree about a moral issue there often seem to be strict limits to what rational argument between them can achieve: each of them may eventually have to cease trying to convince the other person, by baldly asserting a viewpoint which the other rejects, and which cannot be defended by an appeal to anything more basic. Consider, for example, a disagreement concerning abortion: suppose this time that Jane believes that abortion is always wrong, whereas Peter holds that a pregnant woman has no duty to continue carrying her child if this should seriously inconvenience her. This exchange could easily develop into a "dialogue of the deaf", with Jane baldly asserting that innocent human life is sacred and Peter proclaiming equally baldly that every woman may do whatever she likes with her own body. In this case there would be no common ground between the two disputants on the basis of which they might push their argument further. So, having arrived at this state of total disagreement, there they would stick: their discord would be irresoluble by means of rational argument. The problem is, then, that moral disagreements are irresoluble unless the parties to the argument agree in holding certain basic moral principles, such as the principle that innocent human life may never deliberately be taken; but if they disagree about these basic principles, no rational resolution of the disagreement will be possible.

This feature of moral disagreements is certainly evident in many ethical problems arising in nursing. If arguments about basic issues of morality cannot be rationally resolved, what is a nurse to do when she finds herself embroiled in an ethical argument which appears to be intractable precisely because it involves disagreement at this very basic level? Possibly she will be tempted to resolve the conflict in her own mind by arguing in the following way: "Since it seems impossible to show conclusively that my own moral outlook is true and opposing outlooks false, surely I have no right to insist that my personal moral beliefs should prevail when they happen to conflict with the opinions of others? Should I attempt to "push" my views when I know that other people think differently? Would it not be better to accept that everyone should do what he thinks is right?"

The fact that fundamental moral beliefs may seem to lack any solid rational grounding may, then, lead us to adopt a thorough-going type of *moral pluralism*, just as we also commonly favour pluralism in other areas where people's beliefs and tastes differ, such as religion and music and literature. But one who reflects on the apparent groundlessness of moral beliefs may be led to an even more radical conclusion. For, he may argue, if moral beliefs cannot be decisively justified then it is doubtful whether there really are any truths of morality. May it not be that people are simply mistaken when they assert that certain human acts are right and certain others wrong? Could it be that *nothing* is good or bad, right or wrong in itself and that the fact that we think otherwise means only that we are suffering from a kind of systematic illusion? Someone who thinks in this way will naturally conclude, not only that he has no grounds for "pushing" his own moral convictions, but that he has no sound reasons for having any moral convictions at all. And a nurse who consistently adopts that outlook will presumably see her professional work not as possessing any moral significance, but only as a provision of services which other people happen to want and for which her employers are prepared to pay.

We must, then, face the fact that moral beliefs appear to many people to be groundless, and ask: Are they *really* groundless? Or is there some justification for fundamental moral beliefs which a superficial investigation would overlook? If so, does this grounding of moral beliefs and judgments enable us to claim that someone who says (e.g.) "Treating human beings as objects of scientific experimentation is immoral" is saying something which may be objectively true? These questions will be investigated at some length in this and the following two chapters.

The idea of objectivity

The phrase "the objectivity of moral beliefs and judgments", as it is being used here, signifies two things, namely (1) that such beliefs and judgments can be literally true or false, and (2) that they are true or false because of the nature of the human act or acts which they are *about*. Someone could, then, deny this objectivity by denying that either of these supposed features of moral beliefs and judgments really does belong to them. That is, he could, in the first place, deny that moral judgments are capable of being true or false; or, secondly, while conceding that they can be true or false, he could claim that they say nothing about human acts themselves, but simply describe the speaker's attitude towards those acts. We may call the view that there are objective moral truths the objectivist view of morality; by contrast, each of the two opposed positions may appropriately be called a subjectivist view. Let us look briefly at these two different forms of subjectivism.

First, we have the denial that moral beliefs and judgments are ever true or false. This version of subjectivism typically runs as follows. Suppose that a child greets the appearance of his pudding with a cry of "Strawberries and cream – hooray!". In acting in this way, the child expresses his pleasure at the prospect of eating strawberries and cream, but he does not actually state *that* he is pleased at this prospect. Likewise, it is suggested, someone who says "Human experimentation is immoral", or "All abortion is wrong" does not state or report that he disapproves of human experimentation or abortion; rather, he expresses, or gives vent to, his feelings of disapproval. If this view of morality is correct, nothing is ever really, in itself, good or bad, and hence in all the moral difficulties which a nurse may face there is no genuinely right or wrong action.

According to the second form of subjectivism, someone who expresses a moral viewpoint is reporting his own moral attitude concerning the issue in question. On this view, if I say "Suicide is always wrong", I am really saying "I disapprove of all acts of suicide". If I do indeed disapprove of suicide, then what I say is true. If, on the other hand, I have no objection to suicide but am (e.g.) telling a lie because I am reluctant to give my honest opinion, then what I say is false. So this brand of subjectivism treats our moral beliefs and judgments as genuinely true or false, but denies that they make any assertion about the nature of those acts, such as suicide or abortion or truth-telling, which they are ostensibly about. Rather, these beliefs and judgments report my own moral attitudes, of approval or disapproval or, perhaps, indifference, to such acts. Clearly this type of subjectivism is very different from the first type, according to which moral judgments are not true at all. In a sense, however, both subjectivist doctrines come to the same thing; for they both deny that certain kinds of human act are good or bad, right or wrong *in themselves*, regardless of what people happen to think about them.

The first type of subjectivism has traditionally been called "the emotive theory of ethics", or simply "emotivism" – an appropriate title, because it amounts to viewing moral "beliefs" or "judgments" as the projection of emotional attitudes (of approval or disapproval, of satisfaction or disgust, etc.) on human acts. The second viewpoint is more difficult to label conveniently. Since a form of this theory is suggested by some remarks of the Scottish philosopher David Hume (1711–1776), it could, perhaps, be called "the Humean theory". However, the sketchiness of Hume's remarks makes it doubtful whether he fully accepted this theory.[1] No convenient single term suggests itself here, so I shall coin the title "the subjective-report theory". This is an accurate title for the view under consideration, which is that moral judgments are reports of one's own subjective attitudes.

[1] Cf. Hume's remarks in his *Treatise of Human Nature* ed. L. A. Selby-Bigge (Oxford, 1951), Book III, part I, pp. 468–9 ("Of virtue and vice in general"): ". . . when you pronounce any action or character to be vicious, you mean nothing, but that from the constitution of your nature you have a sentiment of blame from the contemplation of it." J. Harrison, in his *Hume's Moral Epistemology* (Oxford, 1976, p. 110), comments that while "Hume sometimes writes as if he held the crude view that to say that an action was wrong or vicious was to make a statement about the feelings [which the act of] contemplating that action aroused *in the person making this judgement*", his more considered view was somewhat more complicated than this.

In this chapter I shall argue that we are forced to give an objectivist account of what moral beliefs and judgments are all about. For this reason I shall criticize and reject emotivism and the subjective-report theory. Both these tasks are evidently indispensable. It needs to be shown that the subjective-report theory is untenable because the belief that rightness and wrongness are real features of human acts themselves appears to be an essential part of what people mean when they say that something is right or wrong. And it also needs to be shown that emotivism is untenable because if none of our moral "judgments" can be true, there is never any obvious rational justification for praising or blaming people for their actions or for inflicting punishment on those whom we call "evildoers". Unless there are what we could call "moral facts", unless our moral judgments can be literally true and say something about things as they are, there is no such thing as morality as it has usually been understood. I shall argue, then, that there *are* moral facts and that what we take to be moral judgments can be true or false.

Emotivism and the subjective-report theory are being accorded special attention here not because they exhaust the field, so to speak – that is, because no other form of ethical subjectivism is conceivable – for this is certainly not the case. There are two reasons why these theories repay close study. First, they remain the two most natural "moves" available to someone wanting to overthrow ethical objectivism, and one often finds that people with no knowledge of academic philosophy say things about morality which indicate implicit acceptance of one or other of these theories. Secondly, even though it is unlikely that any moral philosopher would nowadays defend either emotivism or the subjective-report theory just as they stand, these theories are by no means *entirely* rejected, and they both contain elements which are taken over and supported by some contemporary philosophers. This is particularly true of emotivism, which was first defended in the English-speaking world in the 1930s and which lives on today in the work of thinkers who would nevertheless not defend it in its original form.[1] So a critical examination of these two

---

[1.] For instance, the position known as "prescriptivism", which has been developed by the Oxford philosopher R. M. Hare, takes over many elements from emotivism and is, in my opinion, vulnerable to some of the same objections as those which (I shall argue shortly) show emotivism to be untenable. For a clear statement by Hare himself of his indebtedness to the founder of the emotive theory, A. J. Ayer, see his article "Philosophy and Practice: Some Issues about War and Peace", in A. P. Griffiths (ed.), *Philosophy and Practice* (Cambridge, 1985), pp. 1–3.

positions, however brief, is well worth the effort involved. Let us take a look first at emotivism and then at the subjective-report theory.

Emotivism

The emotive theory was expounded and defended briefly by the English philosopher A. J. Ayer in his *Language, Truth and Logic* (1936), and then in much greater detail by the American C. L. Stevenson in his *Ethics and Language* (1944). Ayer and Stevenson regarded ethical statements as "factually meaningless" – that is, as in principle incapable of being true or false. But, Ayer and Stevenson added, although moral statements have no factual meaning they are not entirely meaningless, for a sentence such as "Murder is wrong" is intelligible in a way that a random grouping of words, such as "Horse afterwards yellow thirteen", is not. So, they claimed, moral utterances have emotive meaning, that is, they serve to express one's emotional responses to various actions and states of affairs. The principal difference between emotivism and the subjective-report theory is that the latter analyzes moral utterances as *reports* of one's emotional or quasi-emotional reactions towards human actions, and reports can, of course, be true or false. But on the emotive theory one does not, in making a moral utterance, report one's emotional reactions but actually gives vent to them. The difference is analogous to that between saying "I am feeling delighted at this moment" and, on the other hand, shouting "Hooray!": in the first case one reports one's delight, while in the second one does not report it but *expresses* it. Now clearly, if one is feeling delighted, then "I am feeling delighted at this moment" will be true; if not, it will be false. But "Hooray!", since it is not a *report* of what is going on in my consciousness, can never be either true or false, regardless of how I am feeling (although to shout "Hooray!" when one feels no elation at all could be regarded as insincere).

So, the emotivists claimed, when I say "Murder is wrong" I am not (as an objectivist would have it) saying something about the nature of murder; nor am I (as a subjective-report theorist would have it) reporting that I disapprove of murder. Rather, I am expressing, or giving vent to, my disapproval of murder. Ayer and Stevenson went on to say that we engage in moral discourse primarily with a view to influencing the attitudes and behaviour of other people. So, by saying "Stealing is wrong" to someone who was on the point of taking another man's wallet I should not be telling him anything true or false, but should rather be expressing my disapproval of his action. And my intention in speaking out would be to influence him to change his own attitudes towards stealing and thereby to desist from pickpocketing. So moral discourse is essentially a practical instrument for changing other people's attitudes and behaviour.

How does the emotive theory stand up to criticism? Well, we should admit straight away that some things which the emotivists said were unquestionably true and well worth saying. They were, for instance, correct in emphasizing the fact that ethical statements can serve to guide and influence people's attitudes and behaviour. But a careful investigation shows that the emotivist thesis, which, like the subjective-report theory, is meant to be an account of what people actually mean when they say such things as "This is a good deed", "That is my duty", "That is evil", and so on, in fact misrepresents the real meaning of those statements.

First, we need to ask the question: What exactly are the feelings of "approval" and "disapproval" which are said to be expressed in moral utterances? It is surely not good enough to say that they are emotional feelings or reactions; for there are all sorts of emotions, some of them (e.g., those of anger, sorrow, hope and fear) being irrelevant to the present issue. We want to know just what distinguishes those emotions which (according to the emotivist) are expressed in moral utterances from all the others. One thing is certain: approving and disapproving, as the emotivist conceives these attitudes, are quite different from the sorts of ordinary likes and dislikes which we express in sentences such as "I like ice cream" and "I dislike the music of Richard Strauss". For the fact that different people have different tastes concerning such things as diet and reading and music does not of itself lead to conflict: if I enjoy eating cabbage and you dislike it, this does not generate a conflict between us unless perhaps I believe on other grounds (e.g., those of health) that you should change your diet. So as far as mere tastes are concerned we are normally prepared to tolerate widespread differences, to live and let live. The situation concerning moral disagreement is, however, totally different. Suppose that I believe that experimentation on human embryos is wrong while you believe that it is right or at any rate permissible. It is hardly likely that I shall regard our difference as on a par with (say) differing preferences over flavours of ice cream. I may not ever try to convert you to my point of view, but I shall at least feel distinctly uncomfortable about your taking the attitude which you do, and would be much happier if you were to change your mind and come to share my rejection of the practice. Why should this be so? Why should we not be happy to live with moral differences, just as we are to live with differences of taste in music and food? If moral attitudes are expressions of emotion, they differ markedly from all other expressions of emotion. How can we explain this difference? The emotivist cannot answer this question, and must treat the action-guiding character of moral judgments as entirely inexplicable. But someone who accepts an objectivist account of morality will be able to offer an explanation of this action-guiding character, by explaining moral approval and disapproval as essentially bearing upon the character of human actions as they are *in themselves*.

Secondly, the idea that moral judgments are typically expressions of emotion is in any case extremely dubious. For although some people do become emotionally agitated when considering or discussing certain moral problems, this is by no means always or even usually the case. Often we reflect deeply on moral matters while all the time remaining unaffected by any emotional feelings. For instance, one may consider by oneself, or talk over with others, the question of whether a nation at war would ever be justified in using nuclear weapons without experiencing any emotional feelings, however slight.[1]

In any case, if there are no objective grounds for the approval or disapproval which I express in making moral judgments, if what I am engaging in is a mere groundless expression of emotions, why should I expect my words to affect the attitudes and behaviour of other people? Why, indeed, should the fact that I have these attitudes be of any interest to them? Suppose that Peter expresses to Jane his repugnance towards cruelty to children. On the emotivist theory, there is not and cannot be anything intrinsically objectionable about any act of cruelty to children *in itself*. So Peter, in saying "Cruelty to children is wrong", is merely giving vent to an emotional feeling which the thought of cruelty to children tends to arouse in him. But if this is all his statement amounts to, why should Jane take the slightest interest in it? Why should she care about the type of feeling which Peter experiences on these occasions – any more than she would be concerned about his having a sour taste in his mouth, or a tingling sensation in his toes? The mere fact that Peter experiences a certain emotion cannot be reasonably expected to influence the attitudes

---

[1] Cf. the criticism of emotivism on this ground in G. J. Warnock, *Contemporary Moral Philosophy* (London, 1967), pp. 26–27.

of anyone else. The emotivists may well be correct in claiming that when we express our moral attitudes we are (sometimes, at least) attempting to influence other people's attitudes and behaviour, but they can provide no rational explanation for this influence.

Thirdly, if emotivism were correct, we could never meaningfully commend or condemn any action which took place in the past, or in general any action committed or contemplated by an agent who was outside our influence. But people often pass judgment on deeds committed in the past – as, for example, on atrocities against civilians during World War II. So judgments of this kind, which are unquestionably meaningful, have to be written off as meaningless if the emotive theory is accepted.[1]

A *fourth* and final objection concerns the emotivists' claim that our moral statements can in principle be neither true nor false. This claim surely misrepresents our conception of morality; for anyone who sincerely makes a moral judgment inevitably regards his judgment as true. If I sincerely assert the sentence "Cruelty to children is wrong", I am proposing this sentence as expressing something true: I believe that I am saying something about the action of being cruel to children, something about that action as it is in itself: *it* is wrong. So we inevitably regard moral goodness and badness as somehow intrinsic to the things and actions which we judge to be good or bad. Now the emotivist presupposes, on the contrary, that goodness and badness are in no way *in* the things and actions judged to be good or bad, and that consequently there is no question of something's being good or bad independently of some person's expressing a favourable or unfavourable attitude towards it. So the emotivist's analysis of our moral life denies the reality of an essential element in our understanding of it. Hence it misrepresents the meaning of the moral utterances which it purports to be analyzing.

The subjective-report theory

We now turn to the second variety of subjectivism distinguished earlier, the subjective-report theory. Although this theory does not receive any

[1] For a rigorous criticism of the emotive theory on this ground, that it cannot accommodate many kinds of moral judgment, especially judgments about the past, see Brand Blanshard's *Reason and Goodness* (London, 1961), pp. 201–203. The whole of Blanshard's long chapter on emotivism (pp. 194–241) is, indeed, a compelling refutation of the theory.

support from contemporary moral philosophers, it deserves to be discussed because this viewpoint, or something very like it, seems to be implicitly held by many people in the world at large, and also in the worlds of medicine and nursing. In criticizing this theory I am not, therefore, attacking a straw man. Consider the following exchange:

Jane: "Euthanasia is always wrong."

Peter: "No it's not; sometimes, at least, it's right."

If this exchange is interpreted on the basis of the subjective-report theory, it has to be represented in the following way. Jane declares that she disapproves of euthanasia in all circumstances. Peter, on the other hand, states that he approves of euthanasia in at least some circumstances. So when someone says something like "Action X is right" he is to be interpreted as *meaning* "I approve of Action X", while if he says "Action X is wrong" he is to be interpreted as *meaning* "I disapprove of Action X". Now since the meaning of words like "good" and "bad", "right" and "wrong" are to be interpreted in terms of the notions of approving and disapproving, these latter notions must be taken to be basic. So a subjective-report theorist will postulate two basic types of moral attitude, one of approval and the other of disapproval. To say that I believe truth-telling to be right is to say that I approve of truth-telling; to say that I believe cruelty to children to be wrong is to say that I disapprove of cruelty to children. (It would be a mistake, on this view, to analyze things the other way round, and say that "I disapprove of cruelty to children" means "I believe that cruelty to children is wrong"; for the notion of disapproving of something is the basic one, in terms of which the notion of believing something wrong is to be analyzed.) Some writers adopt the technical term "pro-attitude" for "attitude of approval" and "con-attitude" for "attitude of disapproval". If we make use of these terms, and of the symbol "=" to signify "means by definition", we can present the following analyses as representative of the subjective-report theory:

"I believe that action X is morally good [or right]" = "I have a pro-attitude towards X".

I believe that X is morally bad [or wrong]" = "I have a con-attitude towards X".[1]

---

[1] These terms, "pro-attitude" and "con-attitude", were used extensively in D. H. Nowell-Smith's influential book *Ethics* (Harmondsworth, 1954).

Since the notion of a pro- or con-attitude is regarded as basic, that is, as unanalyzable in terms of anything else, there is no place, on this view, for objective truths of morality which are totally independent of people's attitudes of approval and disapproval. An act such as murder is *in itself* neither good nor bad; if someone comes along and calls that act "evil" or "wrong", he is not describing the act as it is in itself, but is rather stating or reporting that he has a con-attitude, an attitude of disapproval, towards it. Certainly he is making a statement, he is saying something which is capable of being true or false, but the statement is about him, not about the act of murder. Is this account of morality tenable?

Suppose again that one person says to another, "Euthanasia is wrong". Would it be reasonable to interpret his statement as meaning "I disapprove of euthanasia"? Surely it would not, because in saying "Euthanasia is wrong", the speaker had meant to say something about euthanasia itself, not about his own moral attitude to euthanasia. It seems intuitively clear that this is so, but there are in any case some simple arguments which show that the subjective-report rendering of this moral claim misrepresents its tenor. First, consider the fact of moral disagreement: Peter says "Euthanasia is sometimes justified", but Jane replies "Euthanasia is always wrong". It is clear that Peter and Jane are contradicting each other, that if one of them is correct the other must be mistaken. But on the subjective-report analysis the exchange between them really amounts to the following:

Peter: "I approve of some acts of euthanasia."

Jane: "I disapprove of all acts of euthanasia."

– and on this interpretation there is no disagreement between them, any more than there would be between two people of whom one liked rhubarb and the other did not.

A subjective-report analysis of ethical statements makes nonsense of ethical agreement just as much as of ethical disagreement. For imagine the following exchange between Jane and another friend, Helen. Jane again says "Euthanasia is wrong", and Helen, unlike Peter, shares this opinion, and so she responds "I agree; Euthanasia is wrong". This exchange would have to be represented as follows:

Jane: "I disapprove of all acts of euthanasia."

Helen: "So do I."

On this interpretation the two friends are no more in agreement than they would have been if each had said: "I have a sprained ankle": Jane makes a statement attributing some condition to herself, Helen then attributes the same condition to herself, but these two separate statements are saying different things: there is no *agreement* between Jane and Helen, because two people can be said to agree only when they each assert that *one and the same* state of affairs holds.

Again, consider the fact of moral uncertainty. Suppose that Peter asks himself, in a mood of genuine uncertainty, "Is human experimentation sometimes right or not?". On the subjective-report theory, his question amounts to: "Do I approve of human experimentation in some circumstances?". But this patently misrepresents the point of Peter's question: clearly, Peter wants to know what attitude he *should* adopt to human experimentation; he is not trying to ascertain what his attitude towards it actually is, because at present he does not have any definite attitude.

These arguments show that any attempt to analyze our moral language along the lines of the subjective-report theory would systematically misrepresent the import of that language. The fact is that when we call something good or bad, right or wrong, we do not mean that we have a feeling of approval or of disapproval towards it. Moral judgments typically purport to be assertions about acts or events or states of affairs in themselves, not about our own attitudes to any act or event or state of affairs.[1]

A note on "error" theories of morality

I have argued that both the emotivist and the subjective-report theories of morality systematically misrepresent the meaning of what we say when we assert that something is good or bad, right or wrong. But an advocate of one of these theories could reply that although his theory fails to render the actual sense of our moral pronouncements, it does render accurately *all that we have a right to mean* in saying what we do. While admitting that

---

[1] A possible alternative version of the subjective-report theory is that "Action X is right" means "The society in which I live approves of X", with a corresponding analysis for "X is wrong". One could easily construct arguments against this revised theory, largely paralleling those which defeat the theory in its original form. Since the construction of these arguments is a straightforward matter, I shall not attempt this task here.

people who engage in moral discussion presuppose that their moral judgments are objectively true, he would claim that this presupposition is erroneous. Someone who responded in this way would, in effect, be not so much explaining morality as explaining it away. He would be claiming that there is no such thing as morality at all, as people naturally understand it. We may call this type of theory an "error theory" of morality, since it amounts to the claim that all those who assert that some action is right or wrong, or that we are morally obliged to do certain things and to refrain from doing certain other things, are fundamentally in error.

This account of morality is so totally at odds with our everyday moral outlook that it is difficult to see how one might go about critically evaluating it. It is as if we had to defend the reliability of our sensory powers against someone who claimed: "We have no reason for denying that everything we think we see, hear and touch is really a hallucination". What reply can we make to the error theorist?

One possible reply is that he has no right to claim that the onus of proof is on his opponent, that it is up to the believer in objective moral truths to show that error theories of morality are mistaken. On the contrary, since the view that moral beliefs and judgments can be true or false is part and parcel of our normal, everyday outlook (as revealed, for instance, in the failure of emotivism and the subjective-report theories to render adequately the meaning of our moral judgments) the onus is surely on him to produce some arguments for rejecting it; if and when he does, we can examine the arguments to see whether they are sound. But there is another, more positive, reply which is open to us. This is that there are a number of human acts which, when we consider them with a clear awareness of what they involve, we can see with certainty to be morally right or wrong. Such acts may be few in number, but they are enormously important, because they can serve as the foundation of an adequate theory of morality; by reflecting on them we can come to see that certain *general principles* of morality are to be held. This argument will be developed in the next two chapters. My strategy in this book, then, is to deal with the error theorist's challenge by forging ahead and outlining what I take to be a defensible account of morality and moral reasoning, one which involves accepting the objective truth of moral beliefs and judgments. If this account is soundly-based, it will be clear that the error theorist cannot justifiably dismiss the claims of morality in the way that he does.[1]

★ ★ ★

This Chapter in Summary

Any attempt to deal with ethical problems in nursing today has to reckon with the challenge posed by the moral pluralism which is widespread in our society. This pluralism can easily give rise to a sceptical attitude towards moral beliefs and an uncertainty about whether, in fact, such beliefs are ever really true or false or only (say) the expression of subjective emotional feelings. The sceptical attitudes which sometimes come to light in people's discussions will often be a rough expression of one of the two subjectivist ethical theories examined in this chapter. These are emotivism and the subjective-report theory. Both these theories can be seen, on analysis, to misrepresent the meanings of our moral statements and therefore to merit rejection. Although the idea that moral beliefs are not objectively true or false is certainly fashionable at present, nobody who ever makes moral claims – and that surely means all of us – can take it seriously. Clearly there is such a thing as moral truth; what we want to find out now is the range of principles on which true moral beliefs are based.

[1.] A well-known and much-discussed recent version of an error theory is J. L. Mackie's *Ethics: Inventing Right and Wrong* (Harmondsworth, 1976). For some brief comments on ways of tackling the error theorist's arguments, see J. M. Finnis's *Fundamentals of Ethics* pp. 56–79, and also J. D. Goldsworthy, "God or Mackie? The Dilemma of Secular Moral Philosophy", in *The American Journal of Jurisprudence*, vol. 30, 1985, pp. 43–78. Note here that any theory of ethics which involves denying that moral judgments can be literally true or false will necessarily be an error theory, since it denies something which is part and parcel of our conception of morality. All contemporary ethical theories on these lines can be replied to along the lines sketched above (*viz*, that *if* the objectivist account of morality to be presented in the coming chapters succeeds, the fact of its success will be sufficient to discredit these theories) and they are also vulnerable to the fourth of the criticisms made against emotivism (see pp. 66-67 above). It is for this reason that I have not tried to examine critically such theories as the "prescriptivism" of R. M. Hare If the argument of this and the following chapters is sound, it will follow that all theories of this type are unacceptable.

CHAPTER FIVE

MORALITY AND THE FLOURISHING OF PERSONS

Since emotivism is unacceptable, we are forced to recognize that people's moral beliefs and judgments are capable of being true or false. Someone who claims that lying is always morally wrong may or may not be confused or careless in his thinking; but he does say something which is objectively either true or false. And, since subjective-report analyses of our moral judgments are untenable, whether someone who says "Lying is always wrong" speaks truly or falsely will depend on the nature of lying itself, not on his own subjective attitude towards lying. This means that human actions are good or bad, right or wrong in themselves and regardless of what people happen to think about them. They are objectively right or wrong; in other words, if they are right their rightness is somehow a real feature of what they are, and similarly if they are wrong. What, then, are those features of a human act which determine whether it is right or wrong? If lying is always wrong, what makes it wrong? If, on the other hand, lying is sometimes justified, what makes it right on those occasions?

This issue, of what it is that makes right actions right and wrong actions wrong, is central in moral philosophy. How should one go about tackling it? In this chapter and the next I shall concentrate on one important idea, that morality for human beings has largely to do with what we could call human well-being or fulfilment or flourishing. The conclusions of this chapter are negative, because, it is argued, some attempts to base morality on human fulfilment or flourishing are untenable; nevertheless, the very inadequacies of these ethical theories enable us to grasp what form an adequate account of morality should take.

Morality and human flourishing

Many ethical theorists, notably Aristotle and St. Thomas Aquinas and their followers in the natural-law tradition, have held that morality has essentially to do with what we might call the *well-being* or *full-being* or *flourishing* of persons. The idea is that man, as a rational creature, is capable of shaping his life in a variety of ways, by making decisions which go to form his dispositions and character. By deciding as he does in his day-to-day life he acts either to fulfil his being as a human person or, alternatively, to impede and frustrate the fulfilment of his nature. For in general, some choices, orientations and ways of living fulfil our nature and certain other ways of living deflect us from our proper fulfilment. Just as a plant which is deprived of water or the necessary trace elements will die or, if it survives, will become a sickly specimen of its type, so, on this view, someone who fails to orientate himself to his real end of human flourishing or full-being will end up as a warped and deprived and therefore "sickly" specimen of humanity. This being so, morally right conduct consists in setting oneself to foster human flourishing, in oneself and in others, in certain appropriate ways. Immoral conduct, on the other hand, consists in acting or intending to act against the flourishing either of oneself or of others.

This idea that human flourishing is centrally important for morality could perhaps be disputed. It might, for instance, be denied that morality is exclusively bound up with the welfare of human beings. For even though the brute animals are not moral agents – it makes no sense to talk of a tadpole or a monkey (say) committing a morally good or evil action – the fact that people who wilfully mistreat animals act wrongly means that morality concerns not just human well-being but the flourishing of other types of being as well. Moreover, a traditional tenet of Christian faith is that there are supra-human, purely spiritual creatures, the angels, who, because they possess understanding and free will, are also moral agents: they can grasp what is right and wrong and act accordingly. Since angels are moral agents, there will be criteria for the moral goodness or badness of their acts, criteria which will not, of course, be centred on *human* well-being. Then again, God Himself, as Christians and other theists view Him, is a moral agent. He differs from men and angels in being supremely and indefectibly good, in being unable ever to act wrongly, but the important point is that since God's supreme goodness is a feature of what He is, a part of His nature, it would be wrong to tie morality too closely to the actions of human beings. The importance of the notion of human flourishing is, therefore, that the promotion of such flourishing is a central concern for the action of human beings. It is not necessarily their sole moral concern, much less the sole concern of any (human or nonhuman) moral agent. Considerations concerning human flourishing are centrally important for working out what sorts of actions it would be right or wrong for *human beings* to perform: the effect of someone's proposed action on his fellow men, as well as on the agent himself, will largely determine whether it would be right or wrong. Admittedly, there will be problems concerning man's treatment of the physical world and especially of the animal creation which will probably be insoluble if we confine our attention to specifically human flourishing. However, as far as the sorts of problems to be dealt with in this book – those which typically arise in modern nursing – are concerned, the promotion of human fulfilment clearly will be all-important. Such institutions as health services, medical practices, hospitals and clinics all exist in order to promote the health of patients; and health is an important part of overall human well-being or fulfilment or flourishing. We may, then, regard considerations concerning human flourishing as fundamentally important.

The nature of human flourishing

What does human flourishing amount to? What is it for a human being to flourish rather than to fail to do so? It might be thought that someone is flourishing or fulfilled if his wants or desires are satisfied, that is, if he is doing what he wants to do and is not being constrained to do something against his wishes. However, this suggestion fails because it is evident that many people want things which do not fulfil them as persons but on the contrary obstruct their genuine fulfilment. There are people who devote much of their lives to such activities as seeking money, fame and status, and engaging in casual sexual encounters, which bring no lasting fulfilment or happiness. Such people may succeed in getting everything they want, but they are not thereby fulfilled as human beings. For some, at least, of their wants are objectively worthless, or even positively harmful.

Perhaps, then, human fulfilment consists in the satisfaction not of a person's wants but of his *needs*; for a need is by definition something whose satisfaction would be a genuine benefit. This suggestion has been taken up by some contemporary ethical theorists, who have attempted to list the basic needs which human beings have, to say what they are needs *for*, and to explain how it is that the same need may, in two different individuals or societies, come to be developed and moulded in such various ways. (To illustrate this last point: all people seem to have a basic tendency to enjoy music, but the sort of musical appreciation which a person will come to have will depend upon the extent to which this innate tendency is encouraged and fostered during his childhood, and the kinds of music to which he has been exposed over the years.[1]) This task of specifying the basic human needs is admittedly difficult: different theorists tend to disagree about the number and nature of basic needs which there are, and also about the method to be used in trying to specify them.

One of the problems here is that the words "basic human need" appear to have two distinct meanings: in one sense a person may need something for its own sake, whereas in another sense he may need something because it is a necessary condition for his possessing something else which is intrinsically good. Consider, for example, such things as money, clothing and shelter. People need these things not for their own sakes but because they are necessary conditions for living a good life. A person who is racked by poverty, or has to live in severely cramped quarters, or is kept awake half the night by loud music, is being deprived of certain necessary conditions for human flourishing. Everyone needs a certain amount of money and living-space and sleep if he is to cárry out those activities which are essentially good: but being fulfilled as a human being does not actually *consist in* having money, or living in reasonably spacious surroundings, or sleeping. We can, then, say that human flourishing consists in having one's basic human needs fulfilled only if by "basic human needs" we mean needs for things which are worthwhile in themselves.

The search for human flourishing is largely a philosophical task, to be tackled by philosophical means, because the help which we can expect from other disciplines is likely to be limited. Admittedly, some psychological research on human motivation is relevant to the quest for the basic human needs, but much work in experimental psychology has to do with impulses or "drives" which are directed only to needs in the necessary-condition sense. For example, some psychologists have postulated "drives" which lead us to flee in situations which are felt as acutely dangerous, but we could hardly say that the act of fleeing from danger was itself a constituent of human flourishing. The intrinsically valuable need which is served by this "drive" is rather that of *living* or *maintaining one's bodily integrity*, or something of this sort. Likewise, there is evidently

---

[1] For a penetrating treatment of the "malleability" of human instincts, see Brand Blanshard's *Reason and Goodness*, Chapter 13.

a "drive" to seek food when one is in need of nourishment, but *eating food* is not an intrinsic need, something needed for its own sake. Rather, the intrinsic need is again *to maintain bodily integrity or health*, towards which eating is a necessary means. Despite the evident value of much psychological work in this area[1] the techniques of experimental psychology are not well adapted to tackle this sort of difficult problem, for such techniques can at best provide us with pointers to the basic intrinsic needs of man, which underlie all our overt behaviour but cannot simply be "read off" from the behaviour itself.

Given these difficulties, one may well feel that the idea of identifying human flourishing by specifying the basic human needs is unlikely to be fruitful and that there should be a simpler, more direct way of discovering what human flourishing consists in. This is in fact what has been argued by several ethical thinkers who have claimed that human flourishing is to be understood in terms of certain *basic human goods*.[2] The idea is that there are certain sorts of human action which are intrinsically good. These types of action can all be engaged or "participated" in in a wide variety of ways, but it is nevertheless the case that all human activities which we recognize as intrinsically valuable can be seen as belonging to one or another of these types, or to some combination of them. We can draw up a list of these basic goods simply by reflecting as carefully and rigorously as we can on what things in our lives are intrinsically good, without having to rely heavily on any scientific or psychological data. Human flourishing, then, is to be explained as a certain kind of "participation in the basic human goods".

What are the basic goods? What are these things which are good in themselves and not merely as means to other things? The following list of seven basic goods is based on the works of those ethical theorists who give basic human goods a central place in morality, but it should be noted that these theorists give lists of basic goods which tend to differ very slightly from one another. The first basic good is that of *life itself, including*

[1.] As, for instance, the work of Abraham Maslow, who singles out certain basic tendencies of human nature, called "needs", of which some – the so-called higher needs, for love, for self-esteem and the esteem of others, and for "self-actualization", that is, the ability to think and act as an independently-minded rational individual – identify some of the human activities which are basically and irreducibly good. Cf. Maslow's work *Motivation and Personality* (New York, 1934).

[2.] See G. G. Grisez, *Fundamental Moral Principles* (the first volume of Grisez's projected four-volume work *The Way of the Lord Jesus*), Chapter Five, pp. 115–140, and J. M. Finnis, *Natural Law and Natural Rights* (Oxford, 1980), Chapters Three and Four, pp. 59–99.

health and physical integrity. Since man is an embodied being, the well-being and proper functioning of his body is a necessary part of his total personal well-being. Just to be alive, to be functioning as a living being, is a good for man, even though his total well-being may be impoverished by all sorts of physical and mental afflictions.

Secondly, we have *knowledge*. The inclination to try to find out the truth about things, to discover what is going on around one, why things are as they are – this inclination is at work in the life of everyone who is capable of thinking and reasoning. We all recognize that to know the truth about things is a good, that to be knowledgeable is to be in an intrinsically better state than to be muddled and confused, even if, by being irredeemably muddled and confused, one could escape many of the vexing day-to-day problems of having to grapple with reality as it is.

The third basic good consists in *performing activities of skilful work and of play*. These are activities in which one engages, either by oneself or together with others, not in order to find out the truth about anything or to realize any other ulterior motive, but simply *for their own sakes*. Hobbies and games come under this heading, as does one's day-to-day work when one treats it not just as a means to earning a living but as an end in itself, something one would want to do even if one were not being paid to do it.

Fourthly, we have the basic good of *being aware of and appreciating beauty* in the world around us and in various human performances. To say this is not to say that one can be fulfilled and happy only if one is familiar with all of Beethoven's string quartets and Shakespeare's tragedies. So-called "works of art" are by no means the only objects in which aesthetic enjoyment can be taken; much more basically there is the appreciation of the beauties of nature, for which one needs no special knowledge or training.

The fifth basic good is that of *friendship*. A person who had no friends, whose dealings with other people were confined to business transactions and other kinds of association for furthering his various interests, would undoubtedly be in a severely deprived condition. To be without friends is to be living an inadequate kind of existence. And this is not merely on account of the material benefits which one's friends may often be able to confer upon one but because having friends is good *in itself*.

The sixth basic good is that of what we might call *rationality in ordering our lives* or, more simply, *practical reasonableness*. This is the good of exercising one's intelligence, one's power to respond intelligently to the practical problems which constantly challenge one to decide what to do. It is the capacity to handle rationally such questions as "What should I do?", "How should I react to this situation?", "How should I order my life?".

The seventh and final one of these basic goods is that of *communion with God*, or *having a right relationship with God*. Widespread belief in the existence of a god or gods is a feature of human societies at all times and places, even though there are individuals or groups of people who doubt or deny the religious convictions of their fellows. A person's religious life is by no means confined to believing that God exists. There is also a concern that oneself and one's fellows be in a right relationship with God, that one be doing what is required if this relationship is to be sustained and strengthened rather than weakened and undermined. Christians have traditionally believed that human beings are by nature orientated to a communion with God which would amount to a fulfilment of man's entire nature: this is what is really meant by the statement in the "Penny Catechism" that the end of man is "to know, love and serve God in this life and to see and enjoy Him forever in heaven".

If the seven types of fundamentally good activity identified here are indeed the basic goods of human nature, then human fulfilment or flourishing will amount to some sort of participation in these goods, some mode of realizing them in our lives. Morality therefore concerns the ways in which we should and should not act with regard to our participation in the basic goods.

Is human flourishing really central to morality?

At this point, however, it could be objected that to centre an ethical theory on the notion of human fulfilment or flourishing is to leave out what is most essential to morality. The objection might run: "All this talk about flourishing is irrelevant to morality, and has to do rather with mere self-indulgence or the amoral enjoyment of life. Morality, surely, is a matter of which actions are morally right or wrong, not about which actions foster or undermine our personal fulfilment. For we are sometimes morally obliged to perform acts which hamper our personal fulfilment (as, e.g., in taking care of an aged parent) or to refrain from performing acts which would enhance our fulfilment (as, e.g., in refusing to steal goods which would genuinely benefit us). So the quest for personal fulfilment or flourishing, on the one hand, and the quest for moral integrity, on the other, are totally distinct, and the first of them should always be subordinated to the second: we may seek our own personal flourishing, but only insofar as obedience to moral principles allows. Moral principles, then, are in no way determined by the quest for fulfilment; on the contrary, moral principles place severe limits on what we may do to achieve fulfilment."

This objection has something to be said for it, because there undoubtedly are ways of promoting human flourishing or well-being – either one's own or other people's – which are immoral. For this reason we cannot say just that morally right action consists in promoting human flourishing; something more must be added. But our objector appears to be going to the extreme of saying that morality has nothing to do with flourishing at all, and this is a mistake. For if these two notions were totally separate, it would make good sense to assert that an action which affects human beings but in no way promotes or fosters their well-being is morally good; but the following example indicates that this is not the case.[1] Suppose someone claims that the act of clasping one's hands together is an intrinsically good act, and indeed that everyone is morally obliged to perform this act at regular intervals every day. We would surely reject this claim on the grounds that clasping one's hands together contributes in no way to human good. Only if there were some connexion between hand-clasping and the promotion of human flourishing should we be prepared to take seriously the idea that it might be a worthwhile practice. There would be such a connexion if, for example, hand-clasping exercised one's muscles in a beneficial way; but this is normally not the case. (And even if it were the case, hand-clasping would then be good only as a means, not as an end in itself.) In general, we are never prepared to take seriously someone's assertion that an activity X is morally commendable, a morally good act, unless there are grounds for believing that X somehow contributes to human flourishing. And it is by no means an open question whether X contributes to human flourishing or not. Some activities manifestly do enhance man's well-being; an activity such as hand-clasping evidently does not. So if an act is taken to be morally good, it must be thought to promote human flourishing; and when someone says "X is a morally good act" he is asserting, at least in

---

[1.] This example has been adapted from one given by Mrs. P. Foot in her article "Moral Beliefs", in P. Foot, (ed.), *Theories of Ethics* (Oxford, 1967), pp. 83–100, esp. pp. 90–92.

part, that X helps to promote human flourishing, that it is "good for" someone or other. To say this is not to give the whole truth about morality because, as we have seen, some actions which would promote human flourishing in some ways would nevertheless be immoral. But it is certainly part of the truth: morality, as it concerns human beings, is essentially about *what it is that makes us flourish*. What we want to find is an ethical theory which, basing itself upon this insight that morally good conduct has to do with promoting human flourishing, can formulate criteria for truly judging some human acts morally right and others morally wrong. Is there such a theory?

Utilitarianism

One moral theory which is centred on the promotion of human well-being is utilitarianism. This theory was first explicitly stated by the English philosophers Jeremy Bentham (1748–1832) and James Mill (1773–1836), and then rigorously expounded by the latter's son, John Stuart Mill (1806–1873). Since their time, utilitarianism has been taken over, developed in various ways and defended by many moral philosophers, to the extent that now, at least in some circles in the English-speaking world, it is the accepted orthodoxy. Utilitarianism has penetrated the ways of thought of very many people in our society, from the ordinary man in the street to government ministers.[1] Consider the following clear account of utilitarianism by a contemporary philosopher, J. J. C. Smart:

> . . . the rightness or wrongness of an action depends only on the total goodness or badness of consequences, i.e. on the effect of the action on the welfare of all human beings (or perhaps all sentient beings). . . . [Utilitarianism] is the view that the rightness or wrongness of an action is to be judged by the consequences, good or bad, of the action itself.[2]

---

[1] In a recent survey of attitudes among Anglo-American philosophers, Mr. Bryan Magee observes that utilitarianism "seems to me far and away the most influential moral philosophy in British society today. Whenever Englishmen professionally involved in politics, or the civil service, or any other field of public administration, get together to discuss what to actually do, many if not most of the unspoken assumptions underlying the discussion are those of a rough and ready – often unthought-out – Utilitarianism." (B. Magee, *Men of Ideas* (Oxford, 1982), p. 126.)

[2] J. J. C. Smart, "An outline of a system of utilitarian ethics", in J. J. C. Smart and B. A. O. Williams, *Utilitarianism: For and Against* (Cambridge, 1973), pp. 4, 9.

Suppose, then, that I want to determine whether an action A about which I am deliberating would be right or wrong. I examine the total consequences which would flow from my performing A, and compare them with the total consequences of various possible alternative actions. If the consequences of A are clearly better, in terms of benefiting all those people affected by it, than the consequences of the other possible actions, then I should do A. Otherwise – if one or more of the alternative actions would promote greater all-round human welfare than would A – A would be morally wrong. In general the morally right action is that one which maximizes the possible benefits which I can bring about, not just for myself but for all those affected by my act; a wrong act will be one which falls short of this maximal or optimal benefit. We can see, then, why the utilitarian criterion of morality has traditionally been encapsulated in the formula "the greatest good of the greatest number".

The utilitarian's criterion of right action obviously presupposes that everyone is able to work out and compare the benefits and harms of the various actions open to him. How, then, does one determine whether the consequences of an action are good or bad? What criteria can be used for this purpose? Utilitarians have tended to disagree among themselves on this issue. Bentham and Mill argued that the consequences of actions are good insofar as they involve feelings of pleasure or enjoyment and bad to the extent that they involve feelings of displeasure or pain. This version of utilitarianism has been shown to face serious difficulties, particularly because the pleasure which we take in an action is so closely bound up with the action itself that we cannot prise the two apart and locate all the value in the feeling of pleasure alone.[1] Hence utilitarians nowadays would not make pleasure and pain the criteria of the goodness or badness of consequences. Many of them would be content to say that that action is right which maximizes the fulfilment or satisfaction of people's desires – which, that is, enables the greatest number of people to satisfy their wants or desires or preferences to the greatest possible extent. But since, as we have seen, people's actual desires are often for things which are either worthless or positively harmful, this option is misguided. Only if people's desires are for things which are really good will they be genuinely benefited by having those desires satisfied. To maximize the amount of real good flowing from our actions we shall, then, have to maximize the

---

[1] See, e.g., J. C. B. Gosling, *Pleasure and Desire: The Case for Hedonism Reviewed* (Oxford, 1969), esp. Chapter Three, "Pleasure as a Feeling", pp. 28–53.

fulfilment or satisfaction not of people's mere wants or desires but of their *needs*. And this means (although a utilitarian would not usually put it this way) that the correct action in any situation is that action which brings about the greatest possible overall participation in the basic human goods. Many utilitarians would not subscribe to this formulation, because they are not prepared to recognize that there are real human needs and the corresponding goods, as distinct from felt desires and the apparent goods which they are desires *for*. But it is clear that one cannot identify morally right actions with actions beneficial to all concerned, as utilitarians do, unless there *are* genuinely beneficial actions; and there can be beneficial actions only if people can be truly benefited; and that means, finally, that there are real goods of the human person which correspond to real human needs. So although professed utilitarians would not normally talk about satisfaction of intrinsic needs or participation in the basic goods, one has, I believe, to state the theory in these terms if it is to be at all plausible.

The utilitarian recommends, therefore, that in deciding how to act we should proceed as follows. First, we survey the various alternative actions open to us. Next, we work out, as best we can, the total consequences of our acting in each of these ways for all the people who would be affected. We then compare the various sets of consequences in terms of the aggregate amounts of goodness which they contain. How do we go about assessing the aggregate goodness of the various sets of consequences? Utilitarians would offer differing answers to this question, but the only reasonable answer, surely, is that the amount of goodness in a set of consequences is the amount of satisfaction of human need – that is, of participation in the basic human goods – which it promises. If the choice is between two actions, A and B, and A clearly promises greater overall benefit than B, then, the utilitarian will say, one should opt for A and reject B. So, Smart says:

> Suppose we could know with certainty the total consequences of two alternative actions A and B, and suppose that A and B are the only possible actions open to us. Then in deciding whether we ought to do A or B, [a utilitarian] would ask whether the total consequences of A are better than those of B, or vice versa, or whether the total consequences are equal. That is, he commends A

rather than B if he thinks that the total consequences of A are better than those of B.[1]

Some difficulties in the formulation of utilitarianism

While the central idea of utilitarianism is simple, once we attempt to say exactly what this doctrine amounts to and to apply it to complex moral problems, the going get difficult. One obvious difficulty is that talk about *maximizing* the amount of good obtainable by acting implies that there is maximum good available and that we can discover it by performing the appropriate mental calculation. But neither of these theses is obviously true. Certainly there are some outcomes which we can see to be manifestly better than others: an overall condition of robust good health, for example, is a greater good than an immunity from catching colds. But many choices are made between two or more options of which it is not at all clear which would produce the best outcome. Consider a man who wants to decide how he should leave a sum of £100,000 in his will. The options which he is considering are:

1. Leaving the whole £100,000 to a hospice for the dying;
2. Leaving the whole £100,000 to the Society for the Protection of Unborn Children, so that it can step up its campaign for the repeal of the 1967 Abortion Act;
3. Giving £50,000 to his wife and children, and the other £50,000 to various charities;
4. Leaving £50,000 to his family as before, but with the other £50,000 being donated to his old university; and
5. Passing on the entire £100,000 to his family.

When we consider these five options we see that utilitarian calculation of the greatest overall good is not always straightforward, to put it mildly. Admittedly, if the testator's wife and children have no real need of the

---

[1]   Smart, pp. 13–14. The position outlined by Smart is often called act-utilitarianism, since it asserts that we should do that particular human act which brings about the greatest sum of good consequences. Some utilitarians, however, defend what is known as rule-utilitarianism. According to rule-utilitarianism, an action is right if it is an instance of a general rule (against lying, say, or adultery, or the breaking of promises) and if, by always following that rule, one would produce better overall consequences than one would by trying to calculate, in each individual case, whether to act in accordance with the rule or not. (For a defence of rule-utilitarianism, see J. Rawls, "Two Concepts of Rules", in P. Foot (ed.), *Theories of Ethics*, pp. 144–170.) I have not examined rule-utilitarianism in this chapter because I agree with Smart that when the implications of rule-utilitarianism are fully drawn, it is seen to collapse into act-utilitarianism. (See Smart, pp. 10–12.)

money, the fifth option could *perhaps* be excluded on utilitarian grounds; but otherwise, if the money really would benefit them, it could be that option (5) would do at least as much good as any of the other options. And (1), (2), (3) and (4) could all be considered in the same way, as being perhaps the most beneficial option. If there were a reliable technique for measuring aggregate amounts of good, we could perhaps rank the different amounts liable to be yielded by the various actions open to our testator. But evidently we cannot do this, because there is no such technique. In practice, therefore, the utilitarian's criterion of good and bad action is applicable only in those rare situations in which one possible action is so obviously superior to any other, in terms of the production of good consequences, that no dispute is possible. As far as the many difficult cases are concerned, the utilitarian would probably have to say that if none of the available options is clearly superior to any other, we can treat them as being all equally good – so that *any* of them would qualify as a good or right action, and none of them would be wrong. This option was taken, for instance, by G. E. Moore, who comments:

> [Utilitarianism] recognizes. . . that there may be cases in which no single one of the actions open to the agent can be distinguished as *the* one to do; that in many cases, on the contrary, several different actions may all be equally right; or, in other words, that to say that a man acted rightly does not necessarily imply that, if he had done anything else instead, he would have acted wrongly. . .[1]

But once we make this amendment to the utilitarian criterion of moral goodness, it becomes a much less powerful instrument for moral decision-making than a simple statement of it would lead us to believe.[2]

---

[1]   G. E. Moore, *Ethics* (Oxford, 1912; reprinted 1965), pp. 13–14.

[2]   Some critics of utilitarianism maintain that the different kinds of basic human good are incommensurable, that is, that it makes no sense to speak of one particular combination of participations-in-goods as being "greater" than another. This claim strikes me as questionable, because there certainly seem to be situations in which this sort of comparison can be intelligibly and indeed truly made. (For example, someone's having basic good health and physical vitality is a greater good than his being able to savour different types of wine in a discriminating way – the latter being a mode of participating in the basic good of aesthetic appreciation.) This objection to utilitarianism on grounds of incommensurability is outlined in G. G. Grisez, "Against Consequentialism", in *The American Journal of Jurisprudence*, vol. 23, 1977, pp. 29–141, and J. M. Finnis, *Natural Law and Natural Rights*, pp. 113–116. G. Hallett, in his "The Incommensurability of Values" (in *The Heythrop Journal*, vol. 28, 1987, pp. 373–387), defends the idea that different outcomes of action can be comparatively evaluated and therefore ranked in terms of the goodness which they contain.

Another obvious difficulty is that even before we try to evaluate the consequences of the various acts open to us, we have to determine what those consequences are; and it is usually impossible to do this accurately. The consequences of our acts could be fully predictable if they impinged solely on inanimate objects and had no effect on other human beings, but this is not often the case. Suppose a nurse is trying to decide whether or not she should tell a patient all she knows about his condition. If she is to decide this solely on the basis of consequences, she will have to know exactly how this patient will react to learning this information, how his reaction will affect various other people – his wife, say, and other relations – and how they, in turn, will act as a result. But it is always difficult to predict the reactions of human beings, especially if they are people whom one does not know intimately, and when we are dealing with a whole chain of reactions – of one person on several others, of those others on yet other people, and so on – we are clearly faced with an impossible task. Our actions will typically have consequences extending into the indefinite future and affecting many people who are unknown to us. We cannot, therefore, calculate exactly the *total* consequences of our actions. The utilitarian is, then, obliged to base his judgments of good and evil on what we could call the *reasonably foreseeable* consequences of actions: anything more ambitious than this would surely impose an intolerable burden on our powers of prediction. The notion of reasonably foreseeable consequences is perhaps vague and open to objection, but I shall not pursue this point, since there is, I believe, a more decisive criticism which I shall come to shortly.

Another difficulty arises from the fact that what a person does will affect himself as well as other people, especially if certain actions become habitual for him. So, a man who deliberately kills other people may become a hardened killer; a woman who takes to shoplifting may find that she becomes habituated to this crime and no longer feels any moral scruples about stealing in general. Likewise, a nurse deliberating about whether to lie to a patient about his condition or prospects may worry not only about what effect her lie would have on the patient and his relatives, but also what effect lying would have on herself, on her own moral character. Would her general resistance to lying be weakened, so that she would resort to lies much more easily and frequently? This would amount to a corruption of her own moral character. If utilitarian calculation is to be adequate, it must, then, take into account not only the "external" consequences of my acts, their effects on other people, but also their "internal" consequences, the effects they have on the acting person himself. Somehow or other, these "internal" consequences must be weighed in the balance along with the "external" ones; but it seems clear that this calculation would be extremely difficult and perhaps impossible.[1] This whole issue of the effects which our acts have *on ourselves* will be taken up in Chapter Seven.

A crucial objection

The strong point in favour of utilitarianism is that it takes the consequences of human actions seriously in determining the morality of those acts. This is as it should be, because the probable consequences of proposed actions are indeed important for determining whether they are morally right or wrong. An artillery officer who orders a routine bombardment exercise to proceed even though he knows that some civilians have strayed into the target area acts wrongly, precisely because the artillery barrage could result in their deaths. This sort of example can make utilitarianism seem so obviously true that utilitarians themselves sometimes cannot understand how anyone could possibly reject it.

The recent controversy in Britain over experimentation on human embryos, sparked off largely by the Warnock Committee's recommendation that some such experiments be allowed, illustrates the sort of incomprehension which utilitarians typically feel when confronted by their opponents. The standard argument in favour of experimentation runs as follows: "If embryos are experimented on, we shall learn much about the development of human beings at this very early stage. We shall also be able to detect, very early on, the presence of genetic defects and thereby, we hope, to eliminate these defects from the population. Without this experimental work, however, these benefits will be lost." Here we have a piece of utilitarian argumentation *par excellence*, which many utilitarian moralists would regard as decisive. Consider the following remarks of a newspaper columnist on the Unborn Child (Protection) Bill, which aimed to outlaw all experiments on human embryos and was at that time (1985) before Parliament:

---

[1] See, on this and other grounds of criticism of utilitarianism, B. M. Kiely, S.J., "The Impracticality of Proportionalism", in *Gregorianum*, vol. 66, 1985, pp. 655–686, esp. pp. 666–668.

> On any sane utilitarian calculus, the creation of spare embryos and
> their study in the course of approved *in vitro* programmes will in the
> long term result in more children being born, wanted and
> undamaged. The Bill is not only reductive of human happiness. In
> the ultimate analysis, it is anti-life.[1]

This writer assumes that if some human act is licensed by "a sane
utilitarian calculus" then that is the end of the matter, morally speaking.
But this, of course, is precisely what opponents of utilitarianism would
deny. They would maintain that this is a case in which the consequences
of our proposed actions are not morally decisive. And if we examine the
dispute over embryo experimentation more closely, we see that the
utilitarian's position is not, after all, beyond dispute. For suppose that
human embryos are human beings, human persons in the full sense of that
term, not merely potential human beings. Is it then so clear that it would
be right to experiment on them? Arguments in favour of experimentation
often presuppose that the human embryo, while certainly made up of
specifically human tissue, is yet not a full human being. But if human
embryos are human beings in the full and true sense, differing from the
rest of us only in being radically *immature* specimens of humanity, could
we still approve of destructive experimentation on them?

Suppose, further, that we alter the example so that the experiments are
conducted not on embryos but on five-year-old children. They are, of
course, anaesthetized and have been enticed into the laboratories without
having been caused any apprehension or mental anguish: they do not
know even that they are to be experimented upon, much less that they
will die as a result. Suppose also that these children are orphans and that
their disappearance will cause no-one else to feel any great distress or
sense of loss. Would it be right to experiment on them? A consistent
utilitarian would, I think, have to judge that experimentation would be
right, provided that the benefits promised were sufficiently great. But
surely (we would immediately react by saying) this is wrong: surely it
does not matter whether the research programme involved promises to
produce good results or not; the act of experimenting on and killing these
children would be a grave injustice towards them, a deprivation of their
right to life, which no aggregate yield of good consequences could ever

---

[1]   Geoffrey Robertson, "Go forth and multiply but only if the Minister agrees", in *The
Guardian*, Monday, March 18, 1985.

justify. If this is so, moral problems cannot be solved solely by appeal to consequences.

These reflexions on experimentation on human beings indicate what is, I believe, the clearest and most decisive general objection to utilitarianism. This objection is that a utilitarian who applies his moral theory consistently will be led to approve, and, indeed, to regard as obligatory, acts which we can all recognize with certainty to be immoral.

The crucial premise in this anti-utilitarian argument is that there are some human acts which we know to be intrinsically wrong, just as we know certain basic facts about the physical world, such as: that I am now sitting in a chair, inside a building, holding a pen in my hand, and so on. Admittedly, scepticism about moral knowledge is possible, as is scepticism about the existence of a physical world. But scepticism does not appear to be any more reasonable in the one case than in the other. In the last analysis, the only justification for a belief in morality is that one directly apprehends that certain types of human action are right while certain other types are wrong – just as our only ground for believing in the existence of such things as tables and chairs, human and animal bodies, and so on, is that we apprehend them by means of our senses. Doubtless this assertion of moral truths which are simply "seen" or "apprehended" can appear to be mere dogmatism, sheer groundless assertion. But it would, on the contrary, be mere dogmatism to assert that human knowledge of moral truths was in principle impossible. The only way to test the claim made here is to ask whether there are indeed some instances of certain moral knowledge. The following thought-experiment may be helpful. Consider one of those cases of brutal and sadistic cruelty to young children which are occasionally reported in the newspapers. One's normal reaction is to be seized with horror at the idea that anyone could treat a child in this way, and this feeling of horror includes an attitude of moral revulsion towards the person responsible for the act. Suppose that on such an occasion one explicitly formulates the proposition that torturing children is morally wrong. Can there be any doubt that this proposition is true and that it is immediately apprehended as being true? The answer is surely "Yes": this conclusion, it seems to me, could be denied only if one were in the grip of a general philosophical theory about the nature of reality which (like the logical positivism which underlies emotivism) excludes objective truths of morality.

The argument employed here can be generalized to yield a methodological principle which can guide us not only in rejecting mistaken ethical theories but also in attempting to establish an ethical theory which is correct. The fact is that we do have certain knowledge of some ethical truths, one of which is the truth discussed above, that torturing children is wrong. These truths form the fundamental "data" to which ethical theories must conform if they are to be accepted. (So, a theory such as emotivism which implies that someone who says "Torturing children is wrong" is not saying something true is to be rejected for that very reason.) To a large extent ethical inquiry involves searching for a theory which (1) totally respects the data, and (2) goes some way, at least, towards explaining why the data are as they are. This is why the consideration of destructive experimentation on human beings is important for showing that utilitarianism is mistaken. Once we realize what is really involved in this practice, we realize that it is certainly wrong: this truth becomes part of the data of morality. But it is a datum which utilitarianism cannot accommodate.

One could easily think of many other situations – some real, some imaginary – in which a consistent utilitarian would have to recommend a course of action which we know independently to be wrong. First we have the following imaginary test case, which has been much discussed in recent moral philosophy.[1] In a town in the American Wild West, a terrible crime has been committed, and the townspeople have worked themselves up into a frenzy of protest, demanding that the evildoer be brought to justice. The sheriff knows that there will soon be a riot, probably resulting in several deaths, unless he produces the guilty man – or, at least, a man whom the mob believes to be guilty. He therefore decides to frame, convict and then hang an innocent man. His reasoning is as follows: "I know that this man is innocent, but unless I convict and execute *someone*, far more than one person will be killed. In other words, if I execute this innocent man there will be no further killings, whereas if I let the mob's anger boil over, several other people will die violently. The overall consequences of executing him are clearly better than the consequences of not doing so; therefore I am morally obliged to execute him."

Provided that we make certain assumptions – that the townspeople are unlikely ever to realize the dead man's innocence, that the situation will probably not be repeated, and so on – the sheriff's decision to kill would

---

[1]   See, e.g., the discussion in J. M. Finnis's *Fundamentals of Ethics*, pp. 94–99.

certainly be justified on utilitarian grounds. But in this case utilitarianism must be mistaken, for to kill the innocent man in these circumstances would be wrong. It would be an act of grave injustice against him, which could not be justified by any number of good consequences resulting from his death. This would, I believe, be the verdict of anyone reflecting seriously on this test case, and with a vivid awareness of what it would amount to: anyone whose moral judgments and feelings have not been corrupted will realize that the sheriff's proposed action is immoral, and that any ethical theory which would license it would deserve rejection.

Since this Wild West situation could be thought contrived and remote from everyday life, consider another possible situation, which could easily occur in reality. I have a wealthy aunt who has made me the sole beneficiary of her will. For some time she has been in poor health, although she could live on for some years; and the fact that she is unwell and unable to venture out and about has made her thoroughly miserable. She evidently believes that she has nothing further to live for, and takes little pleasure in any form of diversion. It happens also that I wish to contribute to all sorts of genuinely worthwhile projects, but that I cannot put these plans into effect until I gain my inheritance. There is enormous need for the projects I want to pursue (they include supporting many worthy charities); all that is wanting is money. I therefore decide to kill my aunt by placing poison in her coffee. This action, I say to myself, is not only good but morally obligatory because of the genuine and enormous good which I intend to do by using the money which will come my way and because there is no evil consequence of my act which might count against it.

What would be our reaction to this proposal? I think we should say that the killing would be an immoral deed and that the fact that it would produce benefactions to charity and put an end to my aunt's mental and physical sufferings would be beside the point. Hence, even though, by acting in this way, I should apparently bring about the greatest possible excess of good over bad consequences, the act should still not be done. The fact that a utilitarian would have to recommend such an action indicates the falsity of the utilitarian theory.

As a final example we have a true story, that of Socrates's response to an immoral command by the Thirty Tyrants who ruled Athens briefly after the Peloponnesian War. The Tyrants wanted to execute one of their political opponents, Leon of Salamis, and they ordered Socrates and four others to go to Salamis and bring Leon back for trial. Socrates's reaction was as follows:

> ... the Thirty Commissioners in their turn summoned me and four others to the Round Chamber and instructed us to go and fetch Leon of Salamis from his home for execution..., their object being to implicate as many people as possible in their wickedness. On this occasion, however, I again made it clear not by my words but by my actions that death did not matter to me at all... but that it mattered all the world to me that I should do nothing wrong or wicked... [So,] when we came out of the Round Chamber the other four went off to Salamis and arrested Leon, and I went home. I should probably have been put to death for this, if the government had not fallen soon afterwards.[1]

Since the fall of the Thirty Tyrants could not have been foreseen, it could have been reasonably predicted that if Socrates had co-operated with the plan to liquidate Leon of Salamis better consequences would have been produced than by refusing to do so: for in the first case only one person, Leon, would have been killed, whereas in the second Leon and Socrates would both have died. So on purely utilitarian grounds Socrates would have been morally obliged to assist in the liquidation of Leon. But Socrates was surely correct in claiming that such an act would have been immoral.

The conclusion is that utilitarianism is mistaken, and, more generally, that although the consequences of one's actions for good or ill are often relevant to (and sometimes decisive for) the resolution of moral difficulties, they are not always decisive.

Utilitarians occasionally try to counter arguments of this sort by claiming that utilitarianism is, rightly understood, compatible with the demands of justice. (See, for example, R. M. Hare's comments in *Moral Thinking*, Chapter 8, pp. 130–146.) But such moves on their part usually miss the point of the anti–utilitarian arguments. For example, it is often said that the sheriff who executes an innocent man could never be sure that the truth about his deed would not some day "leak out", with consequences more disastrous than a refusal to take this step. But no

---

[1] Plato, *The Apology of Socrates*, trans. H. Tredinnick, in Plato, *The Last Days of Socrates* (Harmondsworth, 1969); p. 65. See J. M. Finnis's *Fundamentals of Ethics*, pp. 112–120, for a fuller discussion of the anti–utilitarian implications of Socrates's action.

convincing reasons are given for denying the sheriff's ability to keep his secret. In any case, on utilitarian principles it would still be true that *if* the sheriff could be sure that his secret would always remain secure, he would be morally obliged to kill the innocent man; and this is sufficient to discredit utilitarianism.

The principal objection to utilitarianism is, then, that it presents as morally acceptable, and even as obligatory, actions which we know, quite independently of any ethical theorizing, to be immoral. One other objection to utilitarianism deserves a brief mention here, however.

The utilitarian urges us always to perform that action which will *maximize* the flourishing of mankind in general. For instance, G. E. Moore states:

> Our "duty", therefore, can only be defined as that action, which will cause more good to exist in the Universe than any possible alternative. And what is "right" or "morally permissible" only differs from this, as what will *not* cause *less* good than any possible alternative.[1]

But are we really obliged at all times and places to maximize human flourishing? If, after lunch on a summer afternoon, I retire to an armchair to read the newspaper, am I doing the right thing? Only (the utilitarian would say) if I thereby bring about greater total good than by doing anything else – mowing the lawn, collecting money for charity, helping my neighbour with house repairs, and so on. But am I really obliged to make this calculation? Surely, as long as I am not leaving undone some urgent duty, I can read my newspaper with a free conscience even though there are other options available to me which would have produced greater benefit to me and other people. The objection to utilitarianism is, then, that by identifying right action with the *maximization* of good consequences it imposes on people an absurd "obligation" to be perfect. By contrast, Christian moral teaching has traditionally distinguished between those things which must be done or not done as a matter of strict obligation and, on the other hand, further good actions which are "above and beyond the call of duty".[2] The utilitarian's injunction to strive always to achieve the maximum good for mankind in general is impractical and unreasonable.

---

[1] G. E. Moore, *Principia Ethica* (Cambridge, 1903), p. 148.

[2] For a philosophical defence of this distinction which makes no appeal to the data of Christian revelation, see J. O. Urmson, "Saints and Heroes", in J. Feinberg (ed.), *Moral Concepts* (Oxford, 1969), pp. 60–73. See also D. J. B. Hawkins, *Man and Morals* (London, 1960), p. 53.

More – a great deal more – could be said in criticism of utilitarianism; but the criticisms made in this chapter are, I believe, decisive in showing its inadequacy. Is there an alternative theory which can accommodate and to some extent explain the data of morality? If so, how does this theory relate moral right and wrong to human flourishing and participation in the basic goods? This question now requires attention.

★   ★   ★

This Chapter in Summary

Given that some moral claims are objectively true while others are false, the question arises: Can we say what makes such claims true or false? This amounts to asking: Can we say what makes right actions right and wrong actions wrong? One traditional answer to this question is that morality, for human beings, is largely centred on human flourishing or fulfilment or well-being, and that a person's acts will be good if they promote human flourishing in some appropriate way and bad if they either impede or frustrate human flourishing or if, while certainly promoting it, they do so in a way which is wholly *in*appropriate. But this formulation needs to be clarified, because the very notion of human flourishing itself, as well as the distinction between appropriate and inappropriate ways of fostering it, are in some ways imprecise. One attempt to clarify both these notions is offered by *utilitarianism*, which defends the idea that it is the overall maximization of good consequences – "the greatest good of the greatest number" – which is the decisive criterion of some action's being right or wrong. But utilitarianism turns out to be untenable, because it would lead us to approve of actions in which one "does evil that good may come", as St. Paul puts it. While, then, there is much of value in utilitarianism, as a whole it is unacceptable. We need, then, to find an alternative and tenable account of morality and moral judgment.

CHAPTER SIX

IN SEARCH OF FUNDAMENTAL MORAL PRINCIPLES

The aim of this chapter is to defend some basic principles of morality which can be utilized in the chapters to come, when the various kinds of ethical problems arising for nurses are considered. Much of the discussion so far has been a preparation for this attempt to identify the fundamental approach which we should take to moral issues. As far as all this preparatory material is concerned, two points made in the last chapter deserve particular emphasis. These are: first, the importance for morality of the basic human goods, and secondly, the nature of the method to be followed in arguing for or against proposed theories of ethics. A brief recapitulation of these two points may be useful here.

(1) *The basic human goods.*   The morality of human actions is essentially bound up with the flourishing of persons. This flourishing, in turn, can be defined either in terms of the fulfilment of basic human needs or in terms of participation in basic human goods. Either definition could be defended, but I have opted for the second of them, in terms of participation in the basic human goods, since I believe that this goes to the heart of the matter. Human flourishing does consist in the fulfilment of basic human needs, but when we ask what these are needs *for*, we have to answer that they are needs to participate in the basic goods. The word "participation" is justified here, because the basic goods are not particular limited objectives but rather goods which we can realize to a greater or a lesser extent in our lives, and which we can never exhaust, so to speak: no matter how much of a particular good such as knowledge or communion with God we have already realized in our lives, there will always be more – an indefinite amount more – of such realization open to us. The word "participation" is useful also as indicating that the basic goods are not the exclusive property of any one person: we all have the capacity to participate in the basic goods, although the form which such participation takes may differ markedly from one person to another, due to individual differences in terms of innate aptitudes and upbringing, as well as the

ways in which people's characters have been moulded by their deliberate choices and experiences over the years.

It is one thing to say that morality is essentially bound up with the basic goods, and quite another to state exactly *how* the two are connected. Evidently there are certain ways of acting in respect of the basic goods which are appropriate and therefore (morally) right, and certain others which are inappropriate and therefore (morally) wrong. But just how do we distinguish the two ways of acting? Can we state criteria which determine whether some action is appropriate to the basic goods or not? If so, how do we arrive at these criteria? This brings us to the second key point made in Chapter Five, namely:

(2) *The question of method.* The decisive objection to utilitarianism is that it contradicts what I called the "data" of morality. These data comprise various centrally-important truths about the moral rightness or wrongness of certain human acts (either particular acts or general kinds of action) which we are capable of grasping with certainty. There may not be many moral truths of this sort, but there certainly are situations in which the moral rightness or wrongness of an action is so clear as not to be subject to doubt; and a theory of morality, to be acceptable, must be able to accommodate these truths. (In the same way, it is arguable, a theory of human perception must respect the fact that some of our acts of perceiving the world through our senses give us genuine knowledge of what the world is like.) For example, we know that torturing children is wrong, that destructively experimenting on people is wrong, and so on. As the "data" of morality these definitely true propositions can serve as a criterion for the acceptability or otherwise of proposed theories of ethics. For any ethical theory which admits as morally permissible some action which we know independently to be wrong is thereby shown to be mistaken. In attempting to establish a positive account of morality, then, we can appeal to the data of morality in order to correct and refine our formulations of what we take to be the basic moral principles. If we can succeed in doing this, we can then regard our apprehension of those truths which form the data of morality as implicitly based on a grasp of the correct general moral principles which we have isolated.

The basic goods give point and meaning to human life, and participation in these goods is what morality is all about. However, some ways of participating in the basic goods are appropriate and right, while certain other ways of doing so are inappropriate and wrong. If I advance scientific understanding of the causes of genetic conditions by destructively experimenting on young children, I certainly promote my own and other people's participations in the good of knowledge, and perhaps help to enhance the general health of people in my society. If this result alone were required for an action to be morally good, mine would pass with flying colours. What ruins my action, from a moral point of view, is that its beneficial results are bought at the price of destroying the young children who have been experimented upon. Even if the good results of my action should, apparently, totally outweigh the evil of the children's destruction – if, for example, several million people are enormously benefited, as against only half a dozen children destroyed – the action would still be intrinsically evil. So the precise formula we are seeking, which will link morality to the basic goods, will not be anything so simple as (say) "Participation in the basic human goods should be promoted and obstacles to such participation removed", for a formula such as this would admit many actions which are morally wrong. We need something much more specific than this.

What more detailed principle could be suggested? St. Thomas Aquinas formulates the following principle, which he calls "the first principle of practical reasoning": "Good is to be done and evil avoided". I shall interpret this as proposing a specifically moral principle of the kind which we are seeking: this is a natural enough interpretation and is widely accepted, although some recent commentators have argued that St. Thomas did not think of it in this way.[1] Is this principle sufficiently precise for our needs? Evidently not, because it does not itself give us any criteria for deciding what the doing of good and the avoiding of evil consist in. If the doing of good is just a matter of participating somehow in one of the basic goods, then any evil action at all, since it will be motivated ultimately by a desire to realize one or more basic goods in some person's life, will turn out to be acceptable. It could not be excluded by the second half of St. Thomas's principle, that "evil [is to be] avoided", for how could we know that the act was evil? We should have to be given some independent grounds for judging it evil, grounds which St. Thomas's principle itself does not provide.

A recent proposal by the American philosopher Mortimer Adler, aimed at resolving these basic questions, can, I think, be seen as an

---

[1] See, e.g., G. Grisez, "The First Principle of Practical Reason: A Commentary on the *Summa Theologiae*, 1a, q. 94, art. 1", in A. J. P. Kenny (ed.), *Aquinas: A Collection of Critical Essays* (New York, 1969), pp. 340–382.

attempt to give Aquinas's principle the elaboration which it calls for – although Adler bases his proposal on certain remarks of Aristotle in his *Nicomachean Ethics* rather than on Aquinas's deliberations. In addition, Adler works out his moral theory in terms of basic human needs rather than in terms of basic goods, but the role which he gives to basic needs parallels that assigned in this book to the basic goods. For Adler, human beings have certain basic needs which are needs *for* things which really benefit us. Some of the things which people desire or want are largely worthless and bring us no lasting happiness; but

> . . . real goods are the things all of us by nature need, whether or not we consciously desire them as the objects of our acquired wants. Sometimes, as in the case of our biological needs, such as hunger and thirst, our deprivation of the goods needed carries with it pains that drive us consciously to want the food and drink we need. But in the case of other natural needs, such as the need for knowledge, deprivation of the good needed does not carry with it a pain that generates a conscious want for the object of our need. The need exists whether or not we are conscious of it and actually want what we need.
>
> Some things appear good to us *because* we want them, and they have the aspect of the good only at the time that we want them and only to the extent that we want them. In sharp contrast we ought to desire some things *because* we need them, whether we want them or not, and, because we need them, they are really good for us.[1]

Adler goes on to claim that by reflecting on these facts we come to apprehend "a self-evident truth that serves as the first principle of moral philosophy". This is that "We ought to desire whatever is really good for us and nothing else."[2] He believes that this is the only self-evident, underived principle that we need. For we can use it in order to deduce, from premises stating that such-and-such are basic needs of human nature, conclusions about what it would be right or wrong for someone to do in given circumstances. On the face of it this claim is implausible, because Adler's principle, like the one quoted from St. Thomas, is of a high degree of generality. Can something as general as this (we might

---

[1.] Mortimer J. Adler, *Ten Philosophical Mistakes* (New York, 1985), p.125.
[2.] *ibid.*

ask) really enable us to determine the rightness or wrongness of particular human actions? When it comes to illustrating how this principle actually works in moral reasoning, the best that Adler can suggest is the following:

> Starting with the self-evident truth that we ought to desire whatever is really good for us, and adding the descriptive truth that all human beings naturally desire or need knowledge (which is tantamount to saying that knowledge is really good for us), we reach the conclusion that we ought to seek or desire knowledge. . .[1]

Suppose someone acts on this conclusion by seeking knowledge in a way which involves grave harm to other human beings (as, e.g., in destructive experimentation on children). Would Adler's fundamental principle exclude this? Evidently not: it is far too unspecific to rule out an evil action of this kind. Adler needs to introduce some supplementary principles placing limits on the ways in which we are entitled to pursue the satisfaction of our genuine needs; but what those extra principles might be is something of which he gives us no indication.

A theory centred on respect for the basic goods

A more complex moral theory, based in general upon the natural-law ethics of St. Thomas Aquinas, although departing from St. Thomas's stated position in some details, has been developed in recent years by Germain Grisez, and, following his lead, by other thinkers such as John Finnis, Joseph Boyle, William E. May and others.[2] I have already utilized an important part of this theory in listing the basic human goods and in describing our rationally-motivated actions as involving "participation" in the basic goods. Both the classification of the basic goods and the language of "participation" are features of this theory, and I think that what Grisez, Finnis and others have to say in these two areas appears to be true and important: human action *is* centred on our realizing the basic goods in our lives, and this realization *is* appropriately described as

---

[1.] Adler, p. 126.

[2.] Summary expositions of this moral theory are given in J. M. Finnis, *Natural Law and Natural Rights* (Oxford, 1980), Chapters 3–5, and in J. M. Boyle, J. M. Finnis and G. G. Grisez, *Nuclear Deterrence, Morality and Realism* (Oxford, 1987), Chapter 10. The theory is applied specifically to sexual morality in R. Lawler, J. Boyle and W. E. May, *Catholic Sexual Ethics: A Summary, Explanation, and Defence* (Huntington, U.S.A., 1985).

"participation". But these two strands of the theory constitute only its foundational elements or substructure; what makes the theory into a theory of morality is the set of additional elements, the superstructure, which is added on to these foundations. Because this theory of morality has been worked out in detail, it comes much closer than does Adler's theory to explaining why certain kinds of acts are right and certain others wrong. Is this theory completely satisfactory? If it is, we can take it over and use it for our purposes in working out the rights and wrongs of various decisions and interventions in nursing. For convenience I shall refer to this theory as the absolute-respect theory, because it is centred on the claim that people's actions must express an absolute respect for each of the basic human goods. I shall examine the theory principally as it is set out in John Finnis's *Natural Law and Natural Rights*. This is not the most recent presentation of the absolute-respect theory, and Finnis, like other adherents of the theory, has modified it slightly in more recent publications; but this exposition has the great advantage of being very clear and detailed.

Finnis recognizes that the fact that the basic human goods *are* goods, and that participation in them is what constitutes human flourishing, does not by itself add up to a theory of morality. Morality, he points out, enters the picture only when we apprehend a range of what he calls "intermediate moral principles" – so called because they are intermediate between the basic goods, on the one hand, and, on the other, concrete moral norms such as "Adultery is immoral", "It is wrong to kill innocent human beings", and so on.[1] These intermediate moral principles specify the ways in which we should and should not attempt to participate in the basic goods; and from these principles, together with the list of goods, we can deduce the various more concrete moral norms. Finnis believes, for instance, that the Catholic Church's traditional teaching concerning the wrongness of contracepted sexual intercourse can be deduced in this way.[2]

What are these intermediate moral principles? Finnis expounds nine in all. I shall express them in a slightly different order from that which Finnis

---

[1]   Grisez calls these intermediate principles "modes of responsibility" because they are ways of exercising morally responsible choice and action with regard to the basic goods. See *The Way of the Lord Jesus: Basic Moral Principles*, especially Chapter 8.

[2]   J. M. Finnis, "Personal Integrity, Sexual Morality and Responsible Parenthood", in *Anthropos* (Rome), vol. 1, no. 1, 1985, pp. 43–55.

chooses, and as concisely as possible; for a fuller treatment the reader should consult Chapter Five of *Natural Law and Natural Rights*.

First, one should attempt to foster one's own participation in the basic goods in a reasonably systematic way: one should have "a rational plan of life" in accordance with which one's activities are directed. A man would act wrongly if he were to allow himself to be buffeted this way and that by impulses which took his fancy from moment to moment without giving any thought to his longer-term destiny, to what he was making of himself in the long run. To say this is certainly not to say that one must plan the future course of one's life in as much detail as one possibly can; for in view of the vicissitudes of life, any such attempt to put one's future in a strait-jacket would be irrational. All that is required by this first principle is that one have some coherent idea of "where one is going", of the sort of life one is going to lead and hence of the sort of person one is going to be. *Secondly*, given that one has adopted a "rational plan of life" one should take it seriously: for one's future destiny – "what one makes of oneself" – is a serious matter. One should be reasonably strongly committed to the life-plan which one has chosen and should not abandon any part of it lightly. However – and this is the *third* intermediate principle – since even general commitments to lifelong participation in the basic goods can be frustrated by unexpected occurrences, one also needs some flexibility in one's commitment, a certain detachment from particular ways of fulfilling that commitment.

A *fourth* principle is that one should not arbitrarily reject or disregard any of the basic goods. This does not mean that one would act wrongly in having special interests and preferences – by, for instance, cultivating one's musical abilities by regularly practising the violin, at the expense of keeping up with one's friends as one would like. This fourth principle means that even though one cannot give the various basic goods equal prominence in one's life, one must still regard them *as* basic goods, never leaving any one of them out of consideration or deliberately consigning it to a position of no importance in one's life.

A *fifth* principle is that one must recognize the genuine value involved not only in one's own participations in the basic goods but also in those of other people. If I affirm that life, knowledge, play, friendship and so on are basic goods for me, I must, to be consistent, affirm that they are also basic goods for all other beings who share my nature, that is, for all other human beings. The mere fact that I cannot share the conscious thoughts and feelings of other people and am therefore not as strongly motivated to act in their interests as I am to act in my own should not lead me to deny that participation in the basic goods is genuinely valuable for them just as it is for me.

The *sixth* principle incorporates the truth contained in utilitarianism, that one should take account of the probable consequences of one's actions and work efficiently to achieve one's ends. One should strive to "bring about good in the world (in one's own life and the lives of others) by actions that are efficient for their (reasonable) purpose(s). One must not waste one's opportunities by using inefficient methods. One's actions should be judged by their effectiveness, by their fitness for their purpose, by their utility, their consequences."[1] The *seventh* requirement reflects the fact that, as Aristotle put it, man is a social animal. We have a natural concern not only for ourselves but for the whole society in which we live. This requirement, then, is that of "favouring and fostering the common good of one's communities".[2]

The *eighth* principle is that one should not do something which one believes it would be wrong to do. If one has decided that a particular action A is morally wrong, then one would act wrongly in doing A. This will be the case even if one was mistaken in thinking A wrong: the crucial point here is that in opting for A one would be directing oneself towards something believed to be wrong; one would therefore be saying "Yes" to moral evil, consenting to the evil character (as one would believe it to be) of one's action. This moral principle is frequently encapsulated in the slogan: "One should never act against one's conscience." For one's conscience is nothing other than one's capacity to judge that such-and-such a proposed action is or is not morally right. Like all judgments, the judgment of conscience can be mistaken. People's consciences are sometimes described as "sacrosanct", but this must not be taken to mean that what my conscience tells me is right or wrong actually *is* right or wrong. The sentence "A person's conscience is sacrosanct", must be understood as a shorthand form of the view expressed here: a man would act wrongly in going against his conscience, even if it should happen to be mistaken. (It is not implied here that he would act rightly in obeying his conscience, because it could be that his conscience is not only wrong but culpably

---

[1]. Finnis, *Natural Law and Natural Rights*, p. 111.
[2]. *Natural Law and Natural Rights*, p. 125.

wrong – as, for instance, if he has failed to inform himself about relevant facts in which he should have shown interest.)

Finally we have a crucially-important principle which marks this moral theory as belonging squarely in the natural-law tradition and sets it apart from most alternative ethical theories in the English-speaking world in the last few centuries.[1] The principle states that one should never directly attack, or act directly against, a basic human good. An alternative formulation is that "Reason requires that every basic value be at least respected in each and every action", this basic respect excluding any attempt to "choose a single act which *itself* damages and *itself* does not promote some basic good".[2] The idea here is that since human flourishing is a matter of participation in the basic goods, all of which, in a sense, "transcend" us, a certain attitude akin to reverence is appropriate in all our dealings with them. The basic goods are not particular human objectives or results which we could decide to bring about or to prevent, as the mood might take us. Precisely because they provide whatever meaning there is in man's life we must respect them always; and this respect will show itself in a refusal to mount a deliberate and direct attack on any instance of a basic human good. We must, that is, show an absolute *respect* for all the basic human goods in all our actions. One way in which one would fail to respect them would be by attempting to bring about human fulfilment or happiness (one's own or someone else's) by deliberately destroying a person's participation in one of the basic goods. Actions which are directed towards destroying someone's participation in one or other of the basic goods are radically at odds with the respect which is due to those goods, and are therefore not to be done *under any circumstances*.

Consider once again the proposal that one experiment on young children in order to advance the frontiers of medicine and so benefit others in the society and future generations. A consistent utilitarian would have to give his blessing to such a proposal, provided that the predictions of widespread benefit from the experiments were securely based. For what matters to him is the *getting* of good things, the obtaining of good results, and (let us suppose for the sake of argument) some enormously good

---

[1.]   Professor G. E. M. Anscombe has argued that the entire tradition of British ethics in modern times has no place for the idea that there are certain acts which are of their nature evil and so should not be performed whatever the circumstances. See her article "Modern Moral Philosophy", in G. E. M. Anscombe, *Collected Philosophical Papers* (Oxford, 1981), pp. 26–42.

[2.]   Finnis, *Natural Law and Natural Rights*, pp. 120–121.

results are promised by the experiments in question. But if, on the other hand, our attitude is that the basic goods are to be participated or shared in, and are deserving of respect at all times, then our verdict concerning experimentation will change accordingly. We shall say that any treatment of the children in the way suggested would amount to a direct attack or assault on a basic good, the good of life, in the persons of these children and would therefore be evil. Likewise, the sheriff who kills an innocent man in order to forestall a murderous riot acts directly against the good of life in the person of the innocent man and therefore acts wrongly; someone who tells a deliberate lie in order to extricate himself from a tricky situation directly attacks the basic human good of knowledge; a parent who tries to ensure that his child will grow up to be ignorant of all fine literature and music and insensitive to natural beauty attacks the basic good of aesthetic appreciation; and so on. So, in general, it is always wrong to act directly against a basic human good.

If we were to analyze human flourishing in terms of the satisfaction of basic human needs rather than in terms of participation in the basic human goods, it is arguable that we would need to recognize a moral principle corresponding to the one being considered here. This corresponding principle might be, for instance, "It is wrong deliberately to frustrate the satisfaction of a basic human need", or something like that. I do not intend to explore this parallel any further, since the account of moral principles being outlined here is in terms of the basic goods, not basic human needs, but the fact that these two ways of characterizing human flourishing and working out a theory of morality on this basis run parallel to each other is worth noting. A writer who asserts that "Moral evil consists precisely in the frustration of the nature of the agent or those affected by his action," and that "[a moral] obligation arises when otherwise there would be a frustration [of human nature] among the predictable effects of action", is arguably defending a principle running parallel to the one being considered here.[1]

The evil of "attacking basic goods"

The principle that it is always wrong to attack directly any of the basic goods in the person of any human being is of such importance in the absolute-respect theory that it deserves to be called its "master principle".

[1.]   D. J. B. Hawkins, *Nature as the Ethical Norm* (London, 1950), p. 13.

Clearly this "master principle" does, at the very least, contain a good deal of truth. For the basic human goods, since they are basic aspects of the human person, deserve a type of absolute respect appropriate to human persons who are "made in the image and likeness of God". If we take seriously the idea that the basic goods are aspects of persons and not quasi-separable "things" or results of people's actions, it is clear that they cannot be "used" in the way that one would use a physical implement or a plan of action to get what one wants. And if we examine certain kinds of immoral action we can see that what makes them immoral is that they involve using a basic good in precisely this manner. On the surface this is not, perhaps, entirely clear, because the phrase "acting directly against a basic human good" needs to be clarified so that we can determine whether a proposed action would in fact amount to attacking directly a basic good or not. It is arguable that once we do this we can see that actions which are contrary to the principle are morally wrong.

At first sight this is not so, because there are various actions which *seem* to be accurately describable as "attacking a basic human good" but which are obviously morally good. Suppose that the government of a nation declares that because of the death of an esteemed statesman, there is to be a day of mourning, with public games and entertainments forbidden, public houses and children's play parks closed, and so on. Is this government's decree morally wrong as involving an attack on the basic good of play in the persons of the country's citizens? It would surely be unreasonable to say this. If the statesman's death really is a grievous loss for the nation, and therefore something definitely *calling for* deep mourning, it will be right to declare a day of mourning and prohibit games and entertainment on that day.[1] Consider also the following situation. A little girl is playing in her back garden with her toys. Her mother, exasperated because the child has ignored all her calls to come in for lunch, walks out to her and leads her in to the dining room. Has the mother thereby directly attacked the basic good of play in the person of her daughter? If she has, her action would have to be condemned on the absolute-respect theory; but it is surely clear that she does nothing wrong. Again, a man might put an end to a friendship between his daughter and another child whom he judges (rightly, let us suppose) to be likely to lead

---

1.   This proposed counter-example to the "master principle" is presented by Gary M. Atkinson in his "Human Nature as a Ground for Absolute Prohibitions", in *The American Journal of Jurisprudence*, vol. 31, 1986, pp. 137–172, especially pp. 156–160.

his daughter into morally bad habits. Such an action could, surely, be fully justified; but if it amounts to an attack on the basic good of friendship it too runs foul of the moral principle under consideration here.

Any of these three examples could be used as a ground for rejecting the principle which excludes directly attacking a basic good; but it seems more reasonable to deny that any of them involves attacking a basic good at all. This becomes clear if we consider the following parallels to the three cases. A government which prohibits public sport and entertainment, not just on Sundays or on some special occasions but always and everywhere, evidently will act wrongly. Likewise for a parent who deprives his or her child of opportunities for play, not just on certain occasions but over unreasonably long stretches of time. And a parent who prevents his or her child from forming any friendships at all with other children will also act wrongly. In each of these three cases we do have a direct attack on a basic good and hence a morally wrong action. But it is hardly plausible to say that such a direct attack occurs in the original situations, where only a few individual acts of participation in a basic good are suppressed. For basic goods such as knowledge, play, aesthetic appreciation and friendship are goods in which participation or failure to participate is something which takes place regularly, over a period of time, rather than being an instantaneous, all-or-nothing affair. It is therefore reasonable to suppose that one attacks one of these goods not by suppressing it on a single occasion but by suppressing it totally or, at least, unreasonably often. So a mother who never, or hardly ever, permitted her child to play *would* attack the basic good of play in the person of her child and would act immorally. By contrast, an act of lying (for example) is an all-or-nothing affair: in stating something which one knows to be false, one clearly does act against the good of truth, and the fact that most of one's other utterances may be true does not change this in any way. Hence, a single act of lying is a direct attack on a basic good in a way that a single act of suppressing participation in play or knowledge or aesthetic appreciation cannot be.

One of the problems involved in understanding and appraising the absolute-respect theory is that its defenders have done little to clarify the exact meaning of the expression "acting directly against a basic human good" and to determine what kinds of human acts it covers. This is unfortunate, because the expression urgently needs clarification, and there are a number of human acts which appear to be excluded by the principle but are morally right. When, however, we do clarify the principle in the way suggested above, we see that it does not in fact rule out the acts in question. So although, on the face of it, the principle "It is always wrong to attack directly a basic human good" is subject to many counterexamples, most of these clearly turn out on examination not to be genuine counter-examples at all.

However, while this "master principle", suitably clarified, does seem to be true and decisive in ruling out certain human acts as morally wrong, there remains a difficulty about accepting it as applying to *all* human acts. For it could be argued that one of the basic goods, that of life, is an exception to the general rule because there are certain acts of directly attacking this basic good – in other words, deliberately killing a human being – which are morally acceptable. There is, for instance, a long-standing Christian tradition, which finds strong support in people's everyday moral convictions, that while the direct killing by one human being of another is normally a gravely immoral act, there are certain exceptional cases in which deliberate and direct killing is morally justifiable. Among these are:

(1) Capital punishment of those who have committed especially heinous crimes; and

(2) Certain cases of direct killing of combatants (but not noncombatants) in wartime.

If one man kills another, then, it seems, he attacks the basic good of life in the person of the other, because he intentionally brings it about that his victim dies. On the principle we are considering, then, all deliberate killing would seem to be totally excluded. But there is a Christian tradition of support for capital punishment, at least in principle and under certain restricted conditions, which renders any such exclusion untenable.[1] Consider, for instance, the following remarks taken from a popular

---

[1] For a survey of theological teaching on the morality of capital punishment and other types of direct killing, cf. A. Regan, *Thou Shalt Not Kill* (Cork, 1979), Chap. 4, pp. 55–69. Theological reflexion on this subject is based partly on scriptural texts which appear to recognize the justice of capital punishment, such as St. Paul's remarks (Romans 13, 3–4): "If thou wouldst be free from the fear of authority, do right, and thou shalt win its approval; the magistrate is God's minister, working for the good. Only if thou doest wrong, needst thou be afraid; it is not for nothing that he bears the sword; he is God's minister still, to inflict punishment on the wrong-doer." Catholic commentators have traditionally understood this passage, with its reference to the fact that lawful civil authority "bears the sword", as indicating that authority's right to punish by killing.

presentation of the traditional Catholic teaching on capital punishment. In answer to the question "May a Catholic support a campaign for the abolition of the death penalty?", the author, writing before the House of Commons abolished the death penalty in 1965, states:

> ... one must first of all point out that, in any discussion about the abolition of the death penalty, a distinction must be made between the *right* of the State to inflict capital punishment and the *use* of this right. A Catholic may not deny that the State has the right and therefore he may not give his support to any movement for the abolition of the death penalty if such a movement is an expression of the denial that the State has a right to inflict it... A Catholic is entitled to argue, however, that in the present state of our civilization the *use* of the death penalty is not a practical necessity, and to that extent he may give his support to any movement for its abolition which is inspired by humanitarian motives. It must always be understood, however, that even if the use of the death penalty were to be abolished, the State would still have the right, and in a particular case even the duty, to re-introduce the death penalty, if it were to be considered necessary in the circumstances for the security and adequate protection of society.[1]

This passage has been quoted not because it is itself in any way authoritative, but because it does express the traditional teaching of Catholic moralists on this subject. Moreover, the position defended is in no way peculiar to Catholics but is also widely held today by people of all religions and none. Many people, for instance, consider the fact that the State is not permitted to execute the perpetrators of terrorist killings to be a moral outrage. Admittedly, attempts to reintroduce capital punishment in recent years have consistently failed in both Houses of Parliament, but it is arguable that MPs and the Lords are in this respect unrepresentative of their electors and fellow citizens and that if the issue were to be put to a plebiscite there might well be a different result. The essential point, in any case, is that there is this traditional teaching on the legitimacy, in principle, of capital punishment, a teaching which is regarded by many (perhaps most) people in our society as obviously correct; that capital punishment, since it involves deliberately and directly killing a human

---

[1.] J. F. McDonald, *Capital Punishment* (London, 1963), p. 16.

being, apparently amounts to a direct attack on the basic good of life in the person of the executed man; and hence that the Christian moral tradition on this point appears to conflict with the principle that no basic human good may ever be directly attacked. Someone who accepts this tradition may therefore feel forced to conclude that this principle fails to hold universally, that there are some circumstances, even if perhaps very rare, in which such a direct attack could be permissible. Even if it should be established that the traditional Catholic teaching concerning capital punishment is not as authoritative or as securely-based as it has often been thought,[1] the fact remains that the tradition is one of long standing and that it continues to be upheld by very many people who are neither obtuse nor malevolent. This tradition cannot be rejected simply by an appeal to the general prohibition of directly attacking any basic good, because as long as this dispute over the morality of capital punishment remains it is also disputable that the principle really does hold in all cases.

Moralists in the natural-law tradition have generally upheld the principle, not that all killing is wrong, but that the killing of the *innocent* is wrong. This seems to confirm the conclusion that acting directly against the basic good of life may not always be evil; for (the argument would go) one may sometimes, for grave reasons, attack this basic good in the person of one who is not innocent but guilty. A similar conclusion emerges if we consider the direct killing of some combatants in time of war. Clearly this is not an open-ended permission to soldiers to kill whomever they want, as long as their victims are combatants rather than innocent civilians; and normally, since it will be necessary only to disable an enemy soldier, not to kill him, an act of deliberate killing would be wrong. But it could be that bringing about the death of (say) a leading strategist or research scientist working for the enemy side could sometimes be a legitimate military aim, and providing that the war being waged is a just one and that the man selected for killing does indeed play a crucial role in the enemy's war effort, it *could* be that the act of killing him would be justified. After all, because the man is performing a decisive contribution in the service of an unjust cause, he cannot be regarded as "innocent" and therefore as deserving immunity from attack; and the soldier who attempts to kill him acts not as a private individual but as the

---

[1.] As Germain Grisez maintains: see his discussion of killing in *The Way of the Lord Jesus: Basic Moral Principles*, pp. 216–222.

representative of his government, which may be wielding quite legitimately the "power of the sword" of which St. Paul speaks.

This objection to the universal applicability of the principle excluding
any direct attack on a basic human good is worrying because there is no
obvious way of resolving it. Certainly those authors who have developed
and expounded the absolute-respect theory have paid little attention to
this difficulty, and as far as I can tell there is no answer to it to be found in
what they explicitly say. We could try saying that the principle excluding
direct attacks on basic goods applies to all the basic goods *except* that of
life, that the latter is just an exception to it. But this reply would be
unsatisfactory because totally *ad hoc*. Why should there be this exception?
Why should directly taking life sometimes be justified but lying (for
example) never? It could, however, be suggested that although, on the
face of it, a direct killing is always an attack on a basic human good, the
good of life, this is not really the case, or not always. Here considerations
of religious belief enter the picture. The fact is that death is a deeply
mysterious event, and those who believe in the reality of a life after death
have to recognize that they have no accurate conception of what will
really happen at death, of what life after death will be like. For a Christian
this is a matter which he has to leave in the hands of God. But since (on a
Christian view of things) death is not the end of our existence and since
God alone knows what is going to happen to a person, what sort of state
he will be in, after he dies, it *could* be that the killing of a person would not
necessarily be accurately describable as "acting directly against the basic
good of life in his person". At first sight this is hardly plausible, since a
man is a composite of body and soul, and to destroy his body is to destroy
a part of himself and thus really to injure him. But since we do not know
what God has in store for an individual man after death, it is possible, at
least, that death may not count as a genuine injury to him and that the
killing of him is not at attack on the basic good of life in his person.

All this is, admittedly, extremely speculative; but it is speculation
which is naturally provoked by the difficulty of understanding the "master principle" as applied to the basic good of life. Here it is interesting to
note that in Christian moral thought the total rejection of murder and
suicide have often been based not on the fact that they involve directly
attacking the good of life, or intentionally frustrating the fulfilment of
human nature, or anything like that, but rather on the fact that they
amount to an attack on the proper relationship between man and God and
an attempt by a creature to seize for himself the rights of the creator.

For instance, St. Thomas Aquinas condemns suicide on precisely the grounds that

> Life is a gift made to man by God, and it is subject to Him Who is master of death and life. Therefore a person who takes his own life sins against God. . . just as he who usurps judgment in a matter outside his authority also commits a sin. And God alone has authority to decide about life and death, as He declares. . .: "I kill and I make alive".[1]

Likewise, we find a moral theologian condemning the killing of innocent persons on the ground that "when we are dealing with human life – one's own life or the life of another – we are dealing with something in which man can have, at most, only useful dominion." Hence we can rule out "such clear-cut violations of God's absolute dominion as euthanasia and suicide".[2] On this view, the deliberate killing of the innocent is wrong because it involves man's usurping a dominion over the lives of his fellow men which belongs to God alone. This conclusion may be resisted on the grounds that the wrongness of murder is patently obvious to the great bulk of people, unbelievers as well as believers, and so cannot rest on specifically religious premises. But although most people recognize that murder is wrong, they would probably be unable to offer any adequate *reason* for believing it wrong. The suggestion that someone who realizes that murder is wrong bases that belief on an implicit apprehension of man's status as made in the image and likeness of God and subject to God's absolute dominion is not at all unreasonable. Here, it is at least arguable, we can fully understand the rights and wrongs of the matter only if we bring God, and man's relationship to God, explicitly into the picture. Even if one were to deny that the killing of a human being always and necessarily involves attacking the basic good of life in his person, one could still condemn the killing of innocent human beings on the grounds that it amounts to overturning the proper relationship between man and God and thus to attacking the basic good of communion with God.

---

[1] St. T. Aquinas, *Summa Theologiae*, part 2–2, question 64, article 5. The biblical reference is to Deuteronomy 32, 39.

[2] T. J. O'Donnell, *Morals in Medicine* (Westminster, U.S.A., 1960), pp. 55, 60. "Useful dominion" is defined as "that restricted power or prerogative which a man has in regard to another substance whereby he has some right to use the thing, but with certain restrictions which are imposed by the higher rights of others" (p. 54). God, by contrast, has *absolute* dominion over human life.

All these comments and suggestions are, once again, very tentative and speculative. I have made them only because, although the absolute-respect theory does seem to be fundamentally correct and to accord well with the data of morality, it runs into difficulty over the way in which the act of killing is to be morally appraised. The suggestions made here may, perhaps, be of some value for resolving these difficulties. The absolute-respect theory, it is clear, calls out for a rigorous expansion which its authors have so far not succeeded in giving it. But what they have succeeded in giving us is nevertheless immensely valuable.

In the remaining chapters of this book, therefore, I shall attempt to apply the moral principles defended here, and especially the crucially-important principle excluding direct attacks on basic human goods, to various problems raised by nursing practice. The fact that it is difficult to see how this principle is to be applied to problems of life and death, problems in which what is at stake may be the killing of a human being, means that in tackling these problems we shall have to employ a different line of argument. This is the argument based on the contrast between God's absolute dominion over human life and man's purely limited dominion. However, this line of argument itself involves an appeal to the "master principle" which excludes directly attacking a basic good, because when an innocent person is deliberately killed there is a direct attack on the basic good of communion with God. Hence there can be no doubt that this principle is indispensable for dealing with concrete moral problems.

★　★　★

This Chapter in Summary

It is one thing to dismiss inadequate theories of morality such as utilitarianism and another, much more difficult, task to build up an adequate theory which has all the assets of the failed theories, and much more, while avoiding their errors. Such a theory must be founded on the basic human goods, and must succeed in specifying which ways of acting in respect of the basic goods are morally right and which are not. Some attempts to build up an adequate moral theory are clearly faulty, but recent work by a group of moralists who emphasize the idea of absolute respect for the basic goods in all our actions has, at the very least, something to recommend it. A leading tenet of their moral theory is that one must never act directly against any of the basic goods. This principle needs some clarification, especially in the face of possible objections concerning the morality of acting directly against the good of life. It is not easy to see how these objections can be overcome, although various suggestions can be made in this regard. In any case, the immorality of directly killing innocent human beings, as it has been consistently upheld in the Christian tradition, can be defended on the quite separate ground of God's absolute dominion over all life and creation, as against man's essentially limited and derived dominion. In later chapters the moral principles set out and defended in this chapter will be applied to the various ethical problems presented by nursing practice.

CHAPTER SEVEN

MORAL PRINCIPLES, CHARACTER AND INTEGRITY

Among the objections brought against utilitarianism in Chapter Five, one stands out as peculiarly decisive. This objection is that utilitarianism, if taken seriously and applied consistently, would lead us to approve of certain actions which we can see, quite independently of any amount of moral theorizing, to be immoral. We can see that Socrates would have been wrong to co-operate in the liquidation of Leon of Salamis, even though there were good utilitarian reasons for co-operating. Likewise with a sheriff's decision to execute an innocent man in order to forestall a riot which would leave many people dead. As soon as we understand what is involved in cases such as these, we recognize that the proposed action is evil in itself.

This idea that certain acts are intrinsically wrong and therefore under no circumstances to be done runs contrary to most ethical theories popular in the English-speaking world, which assume that nothing is really wrong in itself and that anything at all, no matter how base or repellant it may appear, may sometimes conceivably turn out to be our duty. Most of the philosophers who have made this assumption have failed to recognize explicitly that they have made it, and have tended not to submit it to any critical appraisal. But once we do consider it critically we realize that it is untenable. Historically speaking, the recognition of intrinsically wrong human acts has been bound up with the natural-law tradition of moral theorizing, and in particular with the reflexions of Catholic moral thinkers and the Catholic Church's *magisterium*. So we find Pope Paul VI stressing that "it is never lawful, even for the gravest reasons, to do evil that good may come of it."[1] And more recently Pope John Paul II has

---

[1]   Pope Paul VI, encyclical *Humanae Vitae* (1968), art. 14. The Pope is here echoing the words of St. Paul (Romans 3, 8). It should perhaps be pointed out here that not all Catholic moral theologians are prepared to accept this teaching. As Fr. Richard McCormick says, "Many theologians are arguing that one cannot isolate the object of an act and say that it is wrong in *any* conceivable circumstances." (R. McCormick, SJ, "Notes on Moral Theology 1977", in *Notes on Moral Theology 1965–1980)* (Washington, D.C., 1981), pp. 683–745, at p. 710.

stressed that "there exist acts which, *per se* and in themselves, independently of circumstances, are always seriously wrong by reason of their object. These acts, if carried out with sufficient awareness and freedom, are always gravely sinful."[1]

The view that some actions are evil in themselves and not because of their consequences for good or ill raises issues which centre on a couple of key notions: first of all, the notion of intention, of one's intending to bring about such-and-such effects in acting; and secondly, the notion of moral integrity. The latter notion is obviously important here, for whenever someone realizes that an action open to him would be immoral, he might naturally react by saying, "I couldn't live with myself if I were to do that". Someone who speaks in this way realizes that his moral integrity is at stake, and that this integrity would be shattered if he were to succumb to temptation and do the evil act. The notion of integrity is, then, part and parcel of what we consider morality to be. On the other hand, the idea that one's intentions in acting can crucially determine the morality of one's acts is not so familiar, and may be disputed. I shall therefore consider the importance of intention first, and shall then turn to the connexion between intention on the one hand and integrity and moral character on the other.

The importance of intention

It can be argued that the nature of a person's *intentions* – of what he aims at or sets his heart on, so to speak – is decisive in determining the nature of his actions. For human actions are not just bodily movements, pieces of physical behaviour, but always have a mental side to them as well as a physical side. Hence, two actions carried out with different intentions would be different actions, even if there were no observable difference between the physical behaviour involved in each of them. Consider the action of a doctor in switching off a ventilator which has been keeping a severely-injured patient alive. The doctor may do this because he considers the patient's condition hopeless and judges any continuation of intensive treatment to be pointless. However, he may instead be switching off the machine because, for certain purely personal reasons, he harbours a strong animosity towards the patient and wants him to die. (Imagine, for

---

[1]   Pope John Paul II, Apostolic Exhortation *Reconciliatio et Paenitentia*, 2 December 1984, n. 17 (Vatican translation).

instance, that the doctor's wife had left him and gone to live with this patient.) The outwardly-observable physical behaviour of the doctor may be exactly the same in the two cases, so that in a sense he "does the same thing" in each case. But in another sense he is certainly not doing the same thing, for in the second situation he can be said to kill the patient while in the first he cannot. So a person's action involves not only his observable physical behaviour but also certain mental events and states which underlie and account for his behaviour – in particular, his having certain intentions and certain beliefs about what he is doing.

What a person does is, then, at least in part a matter of what he intends to bring about, what he is aiming at, in behaving as he does. Now a person's intentions are all in some ultimate way motivated by a desire to partici- pate in the basic human goods, because it is the basic goods which give point to all our strivings and activities, even those which are immoral or irrational. So the intention with which one acts will always bear upon participation in the basic goods, either as respecting all of them or as betraying a willingness to attack one or more of them in order to satisfy our desires. If we act with the latter intention, then, as was argued in Chapter Six, we shall be doing something wrong. So morality is largely a matter of what a person sets his heart on, that is, of what attitude he adopts towards the basic goods – and he must take some attitude towards the basic goods because he is engaging with them whenever he does anything at all. Apart, then, from those difficult cases such as capital punishment and warfare which raise some doubt about the *absolute* uni- versality of the principle "Do not act directly against a basic human good", we can say that *if* a person's intention in acting is that someone's participation in one or more of the basic goods be destroyed or curtailed to an unreasonable extent, he acts wrongly. However, sometimes one may act in order to promote someone's participation in one or more of the basic goods, but knowing that one's act will possibly, or even inevitably, result in curtailment or destruction of some other participation or par- ticipations in a basic good. In this case, there is a specifically different kind of act from (say) the deliberate killing of a person, or the deliberate telling of a lie. One's act could not, then, be pronounced immoral as directly attacking one of the basic goods – although it may still be judged wrong on other grounds.

Consider two different situations in which medical teams take action leading to a patient's death.

(1) A medical team who have been treating a grievously-injured road accident victim decide that the case is hopeless, that the man's injuries are too severe and extensive to allow him to recover. They then turn off the life-support systems which had kept him alive, and he dies.

Someone might object to this action on the following grounds: "The surgical team deliberately killed the patient, because if they had maintained life support he would have continued to live for some time. Since the immediate effect of the team's action was the man's death, their action was a direct and deliberate killing of him." There seems to be something wrong here, because this action is surely on a different moral plane from an act of murder. But if so, what distinguishes it from a murderous act? Consider now the second case.

(2) A baby with Down's syndrome is born suffering from duodenal atresia, so that unless he is operated on he will be unable to digest food. Since the child's parents reject him, the paediatrician institutes what is sometimes called a "nursing-care-only" regimen: the baby is kept warm and comfortable, but he is not operated on to remedy the atresia, and he is not fed intravenously, so that eventually he starves to death; and while he is alive he is sedated so that he feels no pangs of hunger.

Suppose that there are no further abnormalities in the baby's condition, that apart from the mongolism and the atresia his physical condition is satisfactory: if, then, the atresia were rectified he would probably live for many more years. Do the paediatrician and the nursing staff directly kill the baby? Surely they do, because the parents and the paediatrician definitely *want the baby dead*, and the hospital team act as they do in order to fulfil this objective: their various actions and omissions are all geared to bringing his death about. Someone might, however, argue that since the hospital team have not actually intervened in any way – e.g., by means of a lethal injection – to end the baby's life but have simply *let him die*, they did not actually kill him. This line of argument would presuppose that the distinction between killing and letting die is morally decisive, and that whereas actively killing someone is immoral, letting someone die does not amount to deliberate killing and is therefore permissible.

Cases (1) and (2) are superficially similar, but if we examine them closely we see that they differ in a crucially important way. For what lay behind the decision not to treat the Downs syndrome baby was clearly *an intention that the baby die*; his parents had rejected him precisely because of his mongolism, and it was decided not to rectify the atresia because that would have enabled him to live. So the steps taken by the paediatrician and the nursing staff were directed towards bringing about the baby's death. As such their action was immoral. By contrast, the decision to terminate life support for the hopelessly-injured patient did not involve any intention that he should die. On the contrary, the medical team wanted the patient to live and would have done whatever was required for this. But they recognized that the case was hopeless, since the patient was inevitably dying. They decided, therefore, that their efforts to keep him alive were pointless, and hence terminated his life support. They accepted that as a result the man would die; but his death was not something they intended to bring about but rather a side-effect of terminating treatment which was pointless.

An objection

Although this idea that a person's intention in acting can determine the morality of his act seems wholly reasonable, not everyone would agree with it. Someone might argue, for instance, that what is important is *what one actually does*, and that one's intention in acting is irrelevant from a moral point of view. Consider any act of the type which we label "doing the right thing for the wrong reason", as, for example, a woman's becoming chairman of her local hospital appeals committee not because she wants to help with fund-raising for the hospital, but because she would, as chairman, be able to bask in the social limelight and attend many enjoyable gatherings. Would this fact alter the rightness or wrongness of the action itself? Not at all, says the objector: the woman's acts as chairman benefit many people in her district and are therefore morally good. The fact that she does these things for an unworthy motive is a sad reflexion on her character, but it remains true that *what she actually does* is good. This is argued, for instance, by Professor James Rachels in his book *The End of Life*. One chapter in the book is entitled "Debunking Irrelevant Distinctions", and Rachels contends that the distinction between acting with a given intention and acting without it is indeed irrelevant, morally speaking. He introduces the following example.

> Jack visits his sick and lonely grandmother, and entertains her for the afternoon. He loves her and his only intention is to cheer her up.

Jill also visits the grandmother, and provides an afternoon's cheer. But Jill's only concern is that the old lady will soon be making her will; Jill wants to be included among the heirs. Jack also knows that his visit might influence the making of the will in his favour, but that is no part of his plan. Thus Jack and Jill do the very same thing – they both spend an afternoon cheering up their sick grandmother – and what they do may have the same consequences, namely influencing the will. But their intentions are quite different.[1]

Rachels claims that since Jack and Jill do the same sort of thing, in the same circumstances, we cannot say that Jack's action was right while Jill's was wrong. Admittedly, Jack's intention was honourable whereas Jill's was not. But "Consistency requires that we assess similar actions similarly. Thus if we are trying to evaluate their *actions*, we must say about one what we say about the other". Rachels continues:

> However, if we are trying to assess Jack's *character*, or Jill's, things are different. Even though their actions were similar, Jack seems admirable for what he did, while Jill does not. What Jill did – comforting an elderly sick relative – was a morally good thing, but we would not think well of her for it because she was only scheming after the money. Jack, on the other hand, did a good thing *and* he did it with an admirable intention. Thus we think well, not only of what Jack did, but of Jack.

> The traditional view says that the intention with which an act is done is relevant to determining whether the act is right. The example of Jack and Jill suggests that, on the contrary, the intention is not relevant to deciding whether the act is right or wrong, but instead it is relevant to assessing the character of the person who does it, which is another thing entirely.[2]

Rachels applies this conclusion to some life-and-death situations in medicine and nursing, in which, on the traditional analysis, two actions, performed with different intentions, would be intrinsically different kinds of action. They are, he claims, nothing of the sort. Suppose that a severely-handicapped newborn baby is examined by two paediatricians. Doctor A believes that deliberate killing is always wrong, but he decides

---

[1] J. Rachels, *The End of Life: Euthanasia and Morality* (Oxford, 1986), p. 93.
[2] *The End of Life*, pp. 93–94.

that this baby's handicaps are so severe that he cannot survive and that palliative care only should be given. Doctor B, who has no such scruples about intentionally terminating human life, decides that the baby could not possibly lead a worthwhile life and that the best outcome for him would be to die as quickly as possible. He recommends palliative care only, precisely in order to bring about the child's early death. Now, Rachels says, since both Doctor A and Doctor B reach the same decision, that palliative care only should be given, they both act in the same way. Therefore the moral quality of their actions is the same: if Doctor A acts rightly, so does Doctor B; if Doctor A's action is wrong, Doctor B's is also.

At first glance, Rachels's arguments are persuasive. For Jack and Jill do seem to be doing the same thing in visiting their grandmother, and the two paediatricians each recommend the same treatment of the handicapped baby. But we need to look more closely here, for it can be argued that Rachels slides over some important distinctions which indicate that intentions are somehow part and parcel of human acts themselves. Consider the following pair of situations. In the first, a French tourist visiting London stops a passer-by and asks the way to Westminster Abbey. The passer-by does not himself know London very well, but he is confident that he knows the way, and directs the man along a street which, in fact, leads right away from the Abbey. The second situation is identical with the first except that the passer-by does, this time, know the way to the Abbey, but out of a hostility to France and the French people he deliberately points the enquirer in the wrong direction. The question is: Do the two passers-by do the same thing in both cases? In a sense they do, because they make the same gestures and say the same words ("You go straight along that road, and you'll see the Abbey after about half a mile.") But surely we can describe their two acts as identical only if we confine our attention to the external behaviour of the two agents in question: once we look beyond this there is a world of difference between the two. Most importantly, one intends to deceive the tourist while the other does not. Hence the two passers-by, despite the superficial similarities of their behaviour, are performing different kinds of action. Here, then, we cannot separate action from intention; the intention actually makes up part of the action. It would be absurd to say here what Rachels says about Jack and Jill, that "the intention is not relevant to deciding whether the act is right or wrong, but instead is relevant to assessing the character of the person who does it". For it is not just that the action of the man who deceived the French tourist must have proceeded from a character which was to that extent bad; rather, his action was itself a bad one.

Why, then, does Rachels's example of Jack and Jill seem to favour the opposite conclusion, that the intention with which an act is performed is totally distinct from the act itself? The answer, I think, is that although Jill regards gaining her inheritance as the *ultimate* goal which her visits to her grandmother are all aimed at achieving, her actual behaviour in the old lady's presence is governed by the intention of giving her a pleasant afternoon. The intention that the inheritance come her way is, so to speak, the commanding, overriding goal which she is striving to attain. But as far as each individual visit to her grandmother and each individual conversation with her are concerned, Jill's intention could well be identical with Jack's, namely, to cheer her up, to afford her some pleasurable moments. She only bothers going to see her grandmother at all because she wants her money; but once she is there she acts towards her with the same intention as Jack does and can therefore be truly said to do the same thing as Jack; and the fact that she has an ulterior motive which is missing in Jack's case does not alter this situation. It is, then, the intentions which are "closest" to Jack's and Jill's behaviour which determine the nature of their respective actions, not the more remote motives or intentions which they might be following, no matter how decisive these more remote motives and intentions might be.

Suppose, however, that Jill is constantly guided by her desire for money in choosing what to say to the old lady: perhaps she regularly lets slip remarks about difficulties in paying for her children's clothes and schooling, her husband's struggle to keep his business afloat, etc. Is it any longer apparent that we are dealing, in Rachels's two situations, with *one and the same* act or range of actions? Evidently not; here, I think we would say, we have two different *acts*: If Jill is all the time conducting herself in her visits to her grandmother with a view to influencing the old lady to change her will in her favour, whereas John is never swayed by any mercenary motive of this type, surely they do not do the same thing, even if (as is most unlikely) the actual content of their remarks should turn out to be fairly similar. So the reason why we feel inclined to accept Rachels's description of the two cases is that we think of Jill's intention to come into an inheritance as prescribing simply that she should visit her grandmother and chat amicably to her for as long as the visit lasts. Jill's intention *while she is talking to her grandmother* is, according to this picture, simply that of giving pleasure to the old lady – and since this is also Jack's intention, it is no wonder that we regard the two grandchildren as doing the same thing.

Rachels is, then, mistaken in denying that a man's intention in acting is part of his act itself and hence that the moral quality of his actions is determined, at least in part, by the nature of his intentions. He is right, however, to see a close link between intention and moral character. It is this link between intention and character which explains the importance of our individual acts for our moral lives. This point needs to be stressed, because some people would object that the only thing that matters, morally speaking, is what changes we actually bring about in the world through our actions. Surely, they might say, when one's intentions make no difference to what actually happens, they cannot really be all that important. It might even be suggested that the concern with intention shown in this chapter is a kind of unhealthy moral fetish, an unreasonable preoccupation with "keeping one's hands clean" at the expense of con-centrating on the doing of good to others. If, however, we reflect on Socrates's reaction to the command to co-operate in the judicial murder of Leon of Salamis, we see that this attitude is unjustified. For Socrates's decision would have made no difference to Leon's fate, and would indeed have cost him his own life if the regime had not fallen. Could it be said, then, that Socrates was unreasonably obsessed with "keeping his hands clean", that his refusal to co-operate with the Tyrants was a kind of unhealthy moral self-indulgence? Would we say this of a sheriff who, out of a determination that justice be done, *refused* to give in to the temptation to frame and execute an innocent man?

The crucial point here is that people's choices inevitably affect their entire characters, that a morally good choice will incline one's character in a good direction whereas a morally evil choice will incline one's character in an evil direction. People sometimes find it difficult to appreciate that this is so, largely, perhaps, because they regard a human act simply as an event which takes place at a certain point in time and is then gone forever. But there is much more to an act of choice than this: it is an act in which one commits oneself to a certain option or range of options; one thereby incorporates these options into one's own character, so to speak; one makes oneself into the kind of person who is disposed to choose in that way. Just as, in general, the way to acquire some habit or ability (the ability to drive a car, for example) is to perform repeatedly the action which one wants to be habitual, so by choosing some option rather than another we deliberately orientate ourselves towards that option and become, more than we were before, the sort of person who favours that option when crucial choices have to be made. Each of a person's successive choices for a given course of action will habituate him more and more towards choosing that act, so that such choices will become more and more "the natural thing to do". This process of habituation may be so decisive that eventually he may find it next to impossible to repent of the choices involved and start out afresh in a new direction. But unless one does repent of the bad choices which have made one's character in part what it is, that character will remain: it will be an enduring part of one's make-up.[1]

In other words, each of a person's acts of choice have what we could call a transitive aspect and also an intransitive aspect. As effecting some change in the world about me, my act has a transitive effect: it "passes over" into the world. But as embodying a commitment which I make in choosing, it has an intransitive aspect because it goes to constitute me for what I am. Suppose I decide to tell a lie in order to extricate myself from some tricky situation. My act of lying evidently possesses these two aspects. Its transitive aspect is precisely its effect on my hearers; if it is successful, they are deceived and I am therefore spared some awkward consequences. But there is an intransitive effect also; for in telling a lie I undermine my own commitment to the truth, I weaken my own orientation to defend the truth and thus make myself more likely to lie when I am tempted in the future. Hence, although the question "What is the agent's intention in acting?" may seem irrelevant to determining the moral goodness or badness of a given action, once we bring into the picture the notions of character and moral integrity and indicate how a person's intentions commit him to certain kinds of action and thus change his character for good or evil, it becomes clear that intention is, after all, morally decisive.

---

[1] For a development of this line of thought, see J. M. Finnis, *Fundamentals of Ethics*, Chapter VI ("Ethics and Our Destiny"), pp. 136–153. Finnis says: "Choices *last*. What choices create is not merely some new wants, preferences, habits. . ., but also a new (not wholly new) identity of character. All free choices last in the sense that they change the person." He adds: "Not that this sort of commitment destroys free choice. One can choose to do what one was committed not to do. . ., by acting unreasonably, inconsistently. . . But one cannot (logically cannot) *escape* from this sort of commitment except by *repenting of* (in a strong sense; not merely regretting) one's former choice." (p. 139.)

The principle of double effect

Since certain sorts of intentions are in themselves wrong and therefore morally corrupting, there will be a crucial moral difference between, on the one hand, intending to bring about some bad state of affairs and, on the other, foreseeing that one's action will have certain bad consequences or side-effects without in any way intending that those consequences should follow. Moralists in the natural-law tradition have attempted to state this distinction rigorously by formulating the *principle of double effect*. This principle is employed to determine when someone may perform an action which will have a "double effect" – that is, two effects or sets of effects, one good and the other bad. It states that it is morally permissible to perform an action with a good effect but also a bad effect if the following four conditions are satisfied:

1. The action in itself is morally good or at least indifferent; it is not itself an evil act.

2. The agent's intention is good. That is, he in no way intends the bad effect; he does not act because he wants to achieve the bad effect.

3. The good effect does not follow from the bad effect. In other words, the bad effect is not used as a means for obtaining the good effect.

4. There is a proportionately grave reason for acting as one does. This means that the good effect which is aimed at is sufficiently worthwhile to justify one's toleration of the bad effect, and that the good desired cannot be obtained without the associated evil or an even worse one.

Moral philosophers and theologians have employed the principle of double effect to resolve many different kinds of problem, but it has been invoked most frequently in debates over medical issues and warfare. Although the principle itself was not fully and explicitly formulated until the nineteenth century, it is implicit in the writings of many of the great Christian thinkers, such as St. Thomas Aquinas.[1] And the fully-formulated principle can be seen as an elaboration of St. Paul's condemnation of "doing evil that good may come".

It could be objected that requirement (3) – that the good effect of one's action not come about through the bad effect – betrays an irrational

---

[1.] See especially St. Thomas's treatment of the morality of killing in self-defence, *Summa Theologiae*, part 2–2, question 64, article 7.

preoccupation with the causal mechanics of events. Someone might ask: Does it really matter whether or not one of the events causes the other, or, if so, which is cause and which effect? But once we see the distinction between cause and side-effect in the light of the intention of the agent, we recognize that it is, after all, morally decisive. Suppose that I want to bring about an event A, but can do this only by first bringing about another event B, from which A will follow. (For instance, I want to bring it about that I inherit my aunt's money, but to achieve this I must first bring about her death, from which my coming into my inheritance will follow.) Then, since I do B as a means to A, it is clear that I intend to do B, even though I intend it only as a means, not an end. If, then, B happens to be evil, in doing B for the sake of A would be "doing evil that good may come". The fact that acting in this way not as an end in itself but as a means to some further end would in no way diminish the immorality of the deed. This third condition of the principle of double effect is, then, entirely reasonable.

Some concrete applications of the principle

A standard application of the principle of double effect is to the case of a pregnant woman with a diseased uterus which must be removed if she is not to die. If the baby she is carrying is viable there is usually no problem: it can be delivered by Caesarian section and the diseased uterus removed. But if the foetus is not viable, the only way of saving the woman's life may be to perform a hysterectomy, which means that the baby will be removed together with the diseased uterus and will inevitably perish. Is it permissible to carry out a hysterectomy under these conditions? The principle of double effect enables us to answer in the affirmative. For the action performed is the removal of the diseased uterus; the baby happens to be inside the uterus, and the operation results in its death, but this should be seen as a foreseen but unintended side-effect of the action of removing the uterus. The mother herself, and the doctors and nurses involved, recognize that the procedure will result in the baby's death but they do not aim at this result. Hence, they do not in any way commit themselves to the baby's destruction, either as an end or as a means. Here the third condition on applying the principle of double effect is crucially important. This condition would be infringed if the baby's death were the means to the removal of the uterus, so that those carrying out the procedure would inevitably act from a death-dealing intention, but this is not the case: the surgeon does not first kill the baby so that he can remove the uterus from the woman's body, but on the contrary removes the uterus, which happens to have the baby inside it. So the performance of the hysterectomy involves no direct attack on the baby being carried, and is therefore justified if there are sufficiently grave reasons for carrying it out. (Here we must keep in mind the fourth condition cited above, that there must be a proportionately grave reason for tolerating the bad effect. This condition would be breached if the good being sought were simply that of avoiding the inconvenience of bringing a child to term. In effect this fourth condition prescribes that the hysterectomy be necessary, or likely to be necessary, to save the woman's life; carrying out the operation for less serious reasons would violate the condition because the reasons for performing it would be disproportionate to the magnitude of the bad effect, namely the death of the unborn child.[1])

Consider another example, this time a military one. A pilot who is fighting in a just cause is attempting to bomb a strategically important bridge. As he approaches the bridge on his bombing run he notices that a child is walking across it. Would it be right for him to bomb the bridge, thereby causing the child's death, or is he morally obliged to abort the bombing run and circle around for another try at it? Let us suppose that anti-aircraft batteries have opened up on the plane, so that any attempt at a second approach would be perilous. Utilizing the principle of double effect, we can conclude that the pilot would act rightly in going through with the bombing raid, even though this would mean the child's death. For the action committed, the bombing of the bridge, is not in itself evil, but (since the bridge is strategically important and the pilot is fighting in a just cause) positively good (Condition 1). Again, the pilot in no way aims at the child's death, either as an end (Condition 2) or as a means (Condition 3). Finally, there is a sufficient reason for the pilot's tolerating the child's death, namely that any second attempt at bombing the bridge

---

1.   The interpretation of the fourth condition which I have given here clearly presupposes that the idea that one state of affairs is a greater or lesser good or evil than another makes sense. This presupposition would be rejected by those natural-law thinkers, such as Germain Grisez, who believe that the basic human goods are incommensurable and hence that different "amounts" of different goods can never be compared in respect of overall goodness or badness. I have not considered this objection because I do not think that this criticism on grounds of incommensurability has been made out. On the contrary, the judgment made above, that the death of a child is a greater evil than the felt inconvenience of bringing a pregnancy to term, seems a clear case of a value-comparison which is perfectly meaningful.

would (because, perhaps, of anti-aircraft fire) be an extremely hazardous undertaking (Condition 4).

The task of expounding and applying the principle of double effect is in sometimes difficult. The discussion of the principle given in this chapter, although necessarily brief, is sufficiently detailed to enable us to employ it in the pages which follow. If the principle is to be properly understood, however, it must be seen in the light of the importance of people's intentions for their possession of moral integrity and for the constitution of their characters. Unless it is viewed in this way, the principle is likely to appear somewhat arbitrary and remote from the real world of moral decision-making. But when the principle is viewed in the light of these crucial facts concerning intention, character and integrity it is seen to make good sense and to cohere well with the facts of our moral life.

Problems of co-operation

An issue which arises regularly in nursing practice is that of *co-operation in evil practices*. Suppose that we are concerned about the morality of a certain practice X, which is normally carried out by at least two people working together, so that it is essentially a co-operative activity: a surgical operation is a clear example. Two important ethical questions can be raised concerning X. First, is X *in itself* a morally wrong procedure? Is the person who carries it out (a surgeon, for instance) doing something evil? Secondly, if X is morally wrong, are nurses and others obliged not to co-operate in any way with those who perform X? Or may a nurse co-operate with them even though she knows that X is wrong? Could she justify her co-operation by claiming that she is *merely* co-operating with someone else's bad action, not performing that bad action herself?

Problems of co-operation arise frequently in such procedures as abortion, sterilization and experimental surgery, where the nurse has to adapt what she does to fit in with the actions of a doctor. In areas such as health visiting where the nurse works largely as an independent practitioner, such problems are likely to arise less frequently. However, nurses can hardly expect to escape these problems entirely. For given that health professionals, like most other people in our pluralistic society, hold widely divergent views about what is right and wrong, a nurse will inevitably face requests for her to co-operate in activities which she regards as evil. She cannot cut herself off completely from what her fellow professionals are doing, and hence she is involved willy-nilly in situations in which (as she believes) bad things are being done. Since there is no possibility of totally escaping involvement in evil, she has to decide where to draw the line. What kinds of evil practice may she rightly involve herself in, and what others should she refuse to countenance?

Suppose that we are concerned with an immoral termination of pregnancy, carried out surgically. (If, as I shall argue in Chapter Thirteen, abortion is in principle an immoral procedure, all abortions are wrong. But all that is being presupposed at the moment is that *some* abortions are definitely immoral.) Precisely because the procedure is immoral, the surgeon who performs it acts wrongly. Likewise, if there is an assistant surgeon who performs part of the operation, he also acts wrongly. But what of the nurses who assist in the operating theatre? They do not themselves perform part of the abortion, and it could therefore be argued that they may be justified in assisting the surgeon. However, since they act as they do in the operating theatre precisely in order to enable him to perform the abortion, surely they they share to some degree in the evil of the surgeon's act.

To deal with these questions we must rely on the conclusions reached already in this chapter, concerning intention, integrity and double effect. Our aim will be to work out some *principles of co-operation* which indicate when co-operation in someone else's evil act might be justified, and when it would be totally excluded.

The decisive criterion here is that of *intention*. A nurse who assists a surgeon to carry out an abortion will have to gear whatever she does in the operating theatre to the goal of having the abortion carried out efficiently and successfully. She will therefore identify herself with the surgeon's intention of carrying out the operation; she will share that evil intention. And since our intentions in acting go to make up our actions themselves, the nurse here, precisely because she shares the surgeon's evil intention, performs an action which is intrinsically evil, just as his is.

It is not only the nurse who assists the surgeon in the operating theatre who shares his intention. If, in handling the patient's pre-medication, or in performing various other activities which prepare the way for the immoral operation, she directs her actions towards the goal of having the operation performed successfully, then, precisely because she acts from an evil intention, she will act wrongly.

The first principle of co-operation which we need to affirm is, then, the following:

Any act of co-operation in another person's immoral action will itself be immoral if the co-operator shares the intention that that action be performed.

The kind of co-operation which is rejected here has traditionally been called *formal* co-operation, since it involves sharing, by intention, in the intrinsic nature or character or form of the evil activity which is being carried out. Hence the principle stated above could be formulated more simply as "All acts of formal co-operation in another person's evil act are immoral."[1]

Suppose, however, that someone co-operates in a way which is not formal, that is, which does not necessarily involve his sharing the intention of one who performs an evil act. Such non-formal co-operation is traditionally called *material* co-operation. Are all acts of material co-operation free from moral objection? No, because the fact that some practice is evil in itself is surely a *prima facie* ground for supposing that one should not co-operate in it. If, then, one were entirely free to pick and choose whether or not to co-operate in someone else's evil act – if there were no compelling reasons for co-operating in it despite its evil character – one would be obliged not to co-operate. The onus of proof, in other words, always rests with the person who co-operates. It is up to him to show that certain conditions obtaining in this particular case justify him in co-operating. In the absence of compelling reasons for co-operation, material co-operation in evil is morally wrong.

What special reasons might justify co-operation? One is that *the co-operation has to be reasonably "remote" from the immoral procedure itself*. The concept of "remoteness" is, of course, somewhat imprecise, and it is difficult to specify just how "remote" a co-operative act must be from the procedure co-operated in if it is to be morally acceptable. Nevertheless, there are situations in which this criterion is clearly enough fulfilled. A nurse who helps in the administrative preparations for a morally objectionable programme of drug trials (assuming that her co-operation amounts to material rather than formal co-operation) co-operates much more closely in the trials than does (say) an electrical technician working

[1.] A similar definition is given in B. Ashley and K. O'Rourke, *Health Care Ethics: A Theological Analysis* (St. Louis, U.S.A., 1981), p. 191: "To actually intend the evil purpose is *formal co-operation*, no matter how small one's share in the actual physical execution [of the evil action]. Advising, counselling, promoting, or condoning an evil action, even when sometimes done merely by being silent when one has a duty to speak up or express an opinion, is formal co-operation because such actions signify agreement with evil."

at the hospital where they are carried out. The technician, just because he helps to keep the hospital operating, co-operates materially in the various procedures carried out there, but his co-operation in the trials is obviously very "remote" by comparison with that of the nurse. Whether the nurse's co-operation will be sufficiently "remote" from the immoral procedure to be justifiable will depend on the actual nature of the contribution which she makes to it, and on how serious an evil the procedure is. If the experimentation involves a grave injustice to patients, it is hard to believe that *any* involvement in administrative preparations for it could be justified.

A second criterion is that the co-operator, by his action, achieves some good result which justifies him in tolerating the contribution which he makes to the evil act being committed. This condition obviously corresponds to the fourth condition on applying the principle of double effect: co-operation is justified only if the end at which one is aiming is sufficiently worthwhile to warrant the co-operation. One may not co-operate in order to gain some good which is not worth gaining at that price, or to avoid some evil which is not worth avoiding at that price. Just what kinds of good might, in fact, be sufficient to justify the toleration of evil which is involved in co-operating will be decidable only by examining individual cases. Clearly the greater the evil which is involved, the greater will have to be the good which is sought if one is to be justified in co-operating. Sometimes the fact that co-operation is required of a nurse as a condition of her employment may be sufficient to justify her in co-operating remotely in certain immoral practices. But if the practices themselves are seriously evil, particularly as involving grave injustice to patients, one could not regard even the keeping of one's job as sufficiently valuable to justify co-operation.

A third criterion for justifying co-operation is that the danger of scandal is avoided, as far as this can reasonably be done. The word "scandal" is here to be understood in the sense common in moral theology, to signify "something that provides occasion and incitement to the sin of another... It is not necessary that sin be actually committed in consequence of it; it is enough that the evil act or word provides incitement to wrong-doing."[1] This criterion is not to be applied to concrete situations in total isolation from the other two criteria. It could be that there are occasions on which one is obliged to tolerate the fact that one's acts give scandal to others, especially if their reactions to one's acts are irrational. But this requirement is to be taken seriously, because the fact that one's material co-operation in evil would give scandal could be sufficient to tip the scales against it and render it morally wrong. Consider the following description by the late Fr. Gerald Kelly, an American moral theologian, of a situation in which there might be "a sufficient reason for permitting a Catholic nurse to remain in a state institution, even though she must occasionally be a material co-operator in illicit operations":

> If nurse Ann leaves this state hospital, she could find work at St. Joseph's Sanitarium. However, at this state hospital she is doing much spiritual good in summoning the priest for Catholic patients, in helping the dying to make their peace with God, in baptizing dying babies, etc. If she is replaced at this hospital by a non-Catholic, this good will not be done.

Fr. Kelly comments:

> We should not be too ready to insist or suggest that Catholic nurses leave public institutions merely because they could get equally good or even better positions elsewhere. The conscientious and exemplary nurse can do much spiritual good in these institutions; and this good more than compensates for occasional and unavoidable material co-operation in evil.[2]

This may well be true if the co-operative acts really are no more than "occasional and unavoidable". If, however, Nurse Ann's co-operation in immoral procedures is required as a more or less regular occurrence, or if she is sometimes required to co-operate materially in acts of grave injustice to patients, it would be impossible to justify her remaining in the

---

[1.] L. G. Miller, "Scandal", in *The New Catholic Encyclopaedia* (New York, 1966), vol. 12, pp. 1112–1113, at p. 1112. The author goes on to quote here the words of Christ in the Gospel: "Temptations to sin are sure to come; but woe to him by whom they come! It would be better for him if a millstone were hung round his neck and he were cast into the sea, than that he should cause one of these little ones to sin." (Luke 17. 1–3, RSV.)

[2.] Gerard Kelly, S. J., *Medico-Moral Problems* (St. Louis, U.S.A., 1959), p. 334.

position. It also needs to be added that considerations of scandal could be decisive here, for Nurse Ann, by remaining in her job and co-operating in various immoral procedures, could influence other nurses or patients to regard these procedures as perfectly acceptable. In this case it would be morally wrong for her to remain in her position, despite the good that she is doing there.

The principles concerning double effect and co-operation set out here are very much general guidelines, and the range and variety of considerations which govern their application to particular ethical difficulties is disconcertingly wide. It may be thought that the general principles are far *too* general to enable us to draw conclusions about the morality of particular acts, or at least to do so with any confidence. But it will become clear in the next few chapters, when we turn to look in more detail at ethical problems arising in different areas of nursing, that this is not so, that the principles do have a good deal of "bite" and can often settle the rights and wrongs of various matters decisively.

★　★　★

This Chapter in Summary

People's intentions in acting can have a part in determining the very nature of their acts: intention is part and parcel of a human act, not something purely "external" to it. Once we realize this we appreciate the force of St. Paul's injunction not to do evil that good may come; and we can also see how considerations of *integrity* can be decisive in moral argument. In the natural-law tradition, the total rejection of doing evil that good may come has been encapsulated in the principle of double effect. This principle, which lays down conditions under which one may act rightly in performing some action possessing a "double effect" – bad as well as good – can be applied extensively to problems of nursing ethics. Problems of co-operation require careful consideration, because even after we have established that a certain practice is immoral, it does not necessarily follow that all kinds of co-operation in that practice are wrong. The traditional distinction between formal and material co-operation can be seen to make good sense and to provide a reasonable criterion for determining which kinds of involvement in someone else's evil act are justifiable and which are not.

CHAPTER EIGHT

TREATING PATIENTS WITH RESPECT

Many ethical problems which arise in nursing come under the heading of "treating people with respect". Of these problems, the most acute concern the nurse's care for her patients. There are, admittedly, problems of dealing with patients' relatives or with other health professionals in which respect for persons is at stake, but since the patient is the focus of the nurse's professional activity, her duty to respect persons will boil down, for the most part, to that of respecting patients. Ethical difficulties centring on respect for persons often lack the dramatic and crisis-ridden character of those concerning abortion, termination of life-support treatment, resuscitation and so on. But problems of this sort are so prominent in nursing that we cannot avoid considering them at some length.

In a sense, the duty to respect patients as persons is an all-encompassing duty; for any sort of harm done to a patient – deliberately killing him or lying to him, for example – will amount to failing to respect him as a person, while many kinds of right action towards him will be describable as "treating him with the respect due to him". But in this chapter I put to one side such issues as those concerning life and death, honesty and confidentiality and so on, and concentrate on problems in which respect for persons is crucially involved and which do not easily fit into any other classification.

In this chapter, then, we focus expressly on respect for persons as beings who have the faculties of reason and will and can therefore think about and order their own lives. Respect for persons as rational and autonomous beings is surely a strict moral obligation for everyone; but problems concerned with treating people with respect seem to arise with particular urgency for health professionals. For patients are often unaware of the nature and extent of their illnesses and depend on doctors and nurses for the information which they want so desperately. Moreover, they may be reluctant to do anything which could be seen as "creating a nuisance", by, for example, insisting on being told the truth. As a result, a patient can be so vividly aware of his own helplessness, and so concerned to receive whatever help is available, that he will accede unquestioningly to any requests made by health professionals. Doctors and nurses therefore have a great deal of power over their patients, and as a result they may be tempted to treat patients with less than the consideration and respect which they deserve. This will apply, above all, to patients who are incompetent, whether through immaturity or through physical or mental illness.

What does "treating people with respect" actually amount to? To treat someone with respect is to treat him as a being possessing intrinsic *value* just because of the kind of being he is. It is to treat him as being valuable in and for himself. Respecting someone is incompatible with treating him as a mere means rather than an end in himself, by *using* him for some purpose or project which one is pursuing. This is what happens when, for example, a medical team conducts research on a patient without his consent, in order to benefit, not that patient himself, but future sufferers from his condition. As some writers put it, this patient is being "instrumentalized", that is, treated not as a human being but as an instrument, something to be *used* by the researchers for their own purposes. Even if these purposes are wholly admirable, this way of treating a patient will be seriously wrong, because it will involve losing sight of the fact that he *is* a human being and treating him as a lower animal or a thing.[1]   Suppose, however, that someone asks: "What is really wrong with using people as means to one's own ends? Why shouldn't I use them in this way if I want to?" How should we answer this question? We might try saying "You shouldn't use other people as you would use an animal or a thing precisely because they're not animals or things." Our questioner may, however, reply: "But what's so special about being a human being? Surely the mere fact that we have various mental abilities which the other animals lack doesn't show that we must treat people in some special way?" After all, it is not always wrong to use something as if it were something else: for example, a book is not a doorstop, but there is nothing immoral about using a heavy volume to keep a door open. Why, then, should the mere fact that man's nature is superior to the natures of animals, plants and inanimate things mean that we must never *treat* a man as we would treat (say) an animal? What if, by using a man as an object of scientific research,

---

[1]   Kant expressed this moral principle in the second formulation of his Categorical Imperative: "Act in such a way that you always treat humanity, whether in your own person or in the person of any other, never simply as a means, but always at the same time as an end." (I. Kant, *Groundwork of the Metaphysic of Morals* Chapter 2, translated by H. J. Paton in *The Moral Law* (London, 1948), p. 91.)

one could acquire knowledge of immense value for the welfare of mankind in general? This seems a powerful objection: if it is wrong to manipulate and use human beings, this cannot simply be because they have certain powers denied to brute animals; we need to show that there is something special about man, something which sets him apart from the rest of the physical world and places him on an entirely different plane from other living creatures. I suspect that we cannot hope to do this unless we bring God explicitly into the picture and say that it is *man's special relationship with God* which renders inappropriate and wrong any attempt to use him as one would use a tool or a brute animal. Given that man is, according to Christian teaching, made "in the image and likeness of God" (Genesis 1, 27), possessing intellect and free choice and destined by God to eternal life in communion with Himself, there is a "sacredness" about man which belongs to no other physical creatures. The fact that man is made in God's image and likeness means that in using a human being as one would a lower creature one is, in a way, attacking God Himself. This is evident, above all, when we consider man not just in terms of his own natural endowments, but as the recipient of supernatural grace which (according to Catholic teaching) elevates him to a condition in which he can – even, to some extent, in this life – share in the life of God Himself. On this view, man has an inherently "holy" character which is foreign to all other embodied creatures; and that demands, correspondingly, that he be treated with the type of respect which we have been describing. As the present Pope says, "the person is the kind of good which does not admit of use and cannot be treated as an object of use and as such the means to an end."[1]

Situations in which respect for persons is at stake

Let us now look at some ways in which the obligation to treat patients with respect is particularly pressing for nurses. Since there are all kinds of

---

[1]   K. Wojtyla (Pope John Paul II), *Love and Responsibility* (London, 1981), p. 41. Some Christian ethicists connect this fact of the "sacred" character of human life with God's becoming incarnate in Jesus Christ: "Every living human body, the one that comes to be when new human life is conceived, is a living image of the all-holy God. Moreover, in creating Man, male and female, God created a being inwardly capable of being divinized. God cannot become incarnate in a pig or ape or dolphin. But, as we know from God's revelation, He can become incarnate in a human creature and in fact has chosen freely to become truly one of us. . . Every human being, therefore, is intrinsically valuable, surpassing in dignity the whole material universe, a being to be revered and respected from the very beginning of its existence." (W. E. May, "Human Dignity: What and Whence?", in *Ethics & Medics*, vol 12, no. 11, November 1987, p. 4.)

ways in which a person can be treated with *dis*respect, the problems we encounter in this area will be immensely varied. I have classified these problems into the following eight subgroups:

1. Treating patients with kindness, courtesy and consideration whenever one is talking to them, or putting them through some examination or prescribed procedure, etc.

2. Providing patients with the treatment and care which they need, and avoiding carelessness and unnecessary delay in attending to these needs.

3. Refraining from using patients for purely experimental purposes or as mere means for the training of doctors and nurses.

4. Obtaining patients' consent for all operations or other forms of treatment.

5. Keeping patients informed about what is going on as far as their courses of treatment are concerned.

6. Respecting patients' beliefs (including their moral and religious beliefs) and cultural background.

7. Caring for unconscious or otherwise incompetent patients.

8. Treating patients who are mentally ill.

This eightfold classification is not absolutely "watertight", and some of the subgroups will inevitably overlap – e.g., (1) and (2), since failing to provide a patient with the nursing care which he needs also amounts to behaving discourteously and inconsiderately towards him. This amount of overlap should not worry us unduly, however, as a classification into completely self-contained compartments is probably unattainable. Let us now consider these eight general problem areas one by one.

(1) Kindness and courtesy to patients

An important expression of concern for people's genuine good is kind and considerate treatment of them. By contrast, rudeness or an off-hand manner naturally expresses indifference or even hostility to the good of others. The nurse's work of caring for people will therefore involve her

treating them kindly and being courteous towards them. This requirement of courtesy and consideration applies, of course, to people in all
walks of life. But it is particularly important for nurses, since they are
dealing with people who are physically and mentally in a vulnerable and
often stressful state.

A nurse who fails to treat patients with kindness and consideration may
act in ways which, while unsatisfactory and wrong, are nevertheless not
too far removed from the correct standard. On the other hand, she may
do something which is grossly at odds with the way she should treat her
patients. There is, in other words, a whole range or spectrum of bad
behaviour, some of it bad but not too bad, while some other instances of
it (e.g., physically assaulting a patient) are grossly immoral and make the
nurse liable to dismissal and to legal action. Instances of abuse and assault
of patients are rare (the latter probably extremely rare, even though it
does happen[1]); and so we can concentrate on the more everyday examples
of unkindness and discourtesy which a nurse (especially one under intense
pressure as a result of demands from patients, etc.) may be prone to
display. Consider the following episode which was reported to me:

> "A male medical patient with cancer of the prostate gland was on a
> synthetic female hormone which had the effect of causing the begin-
> nings of female secondary sex characteristics to appear. This elderly
> man was teased about his 'breasts' by a member of the staff, which
> was a cruel and unkind thing to do."

Probably there was no malicious intent underlying the reported remark.
Rather, there was a lack of consideration for the patient, a thoughtless
over-familiarity with him, a failure to appreciate just how disorientating
this unnatural change in his physical appearance would be. Similarly, a
nurse who presumes to address an adult patient by his first name, even
though he has not asked to be treated with this sort of familiarity, will also
be open to criticism, for putting oneself on first-name terms with patients
who have not requested this is an unjustifiable liberty on the part of a
health professional. This sort of carelessness and inattention to patients'
sensitivities can be avoided only by a real effort on the nurse's part to "get
inside" the minds of her patients, to understand how their conditions are

---

[1]. An example of a particularly reprehensible act is discussed by A. Langslow, in her article
"Age must not invite harm or hurt", in *The Australian Nurses Journal*, vol. 14, no. 6, December
1984/January 1985, p. 20.

likely to affect them and the way they are likely to react if treated in certain ways.

None of these examples of unkind or discourteous behaviour raises any intractable moral problem; for it is clear that the nurse should not treat her patients in these ways, because to do so would be to infringe the patient's inherent dignity simply as a human being. Ethical difficulties do arise, however, when we ask how a nurse should react when she witnesses another nurse treating a patient unkindly or discourteously. Should she react at all? If so, how? There seem to be two possibilities here: the nurse may approach her colleague and point out the impropriety of his or her action, or she may report that colleague to her ward sister or some other, more senior nurse. Probably the first, more restrained approach should be taken to relatively minor infringements of the respect-for-patients requirement, especially if they are isolated incidents and the offending nurse has not made a settled habit of them; whereas the second approach would be appropriate for habitual infringements and, of course, for any action verging on assault. But much will also depend upon the facts of each particular case, such as the personality of the offending nurse and his or her likely reaction if approached and criticized.

Sometimes it is a doctor rather than another nurse who treats a patient inconsiderately, as in the following incident:

"During a round of the maternity ward, we were standing around a patient with chronic renal failure with whom I had become quite friendly. She was very worried about the fact that her labour might soon need to be induced and that she might have to have a caesarian operation. However, the three doctors and three medical students did not seem at all aware of the lady's feelings as they talked at great length of her condition and how they diagnosed it and what they might do. They did not once look at her while talking, and she was a different person to the bright cheerful woman I knew as she nibbled at her neck chain. What shocked me was probably the extreme feeling, which I sensed that she had, of wishing to disappear into non-existence. She seemed so transformed, and it was only at the very end that the consultant turned to her; she seemed merely an object in bed to the six of them."

Because this doctor's attitudes and actions towards the patient were inconsiderate, he was wrong to treat her as he did. But the nurse who witnessed this episode may wonder whether she should try to rectify the situation somehow and/or persuade the doctor to change his attitude in future, or instead to do nothing. The options open to the nurse will depend on many factors. If, for instance, she is a reserved and somewhat timid student nurse, while the consultant has an aura of unapproachability and seems likely to resent criticism, she could not reasonably be expected to approach him about the incident. She may be able to do something *via* her more senior nursing colleagues, or simply by attempting to reassure and comfort the patient. All of these are options, the last one being perhaps the most useful. We find here, as elsewhere in nursing, that no hard-and-fast rules can be laid down; rather, each case has to be treated on the basis of the nurse's own judgment and her sensitivity to other people's attitudes and reactions.

(2) Attending adequately to patients' needs

When a nurse takes on a position in a hospital, medical centre or some other establishment, she implicitly undertakes to provide whatever her patients need for the restoration or maintenance of their health. Clearly the extent to which a nurse will be able to fulfil this requirement will depend on many factors, some of them outside her control. If, for instance, her ward is understaffed she may be unable to attend adequately to patients' needs. But in the absence of these special circumstances a failure to attend to patients' needs will be a culpable moral failure. One serious infringement of this requirement is the failure to give adequate relief of pain, especially for patients who are terminally ill with cancer and who would suffer severe and constant pain without analgesia. A nurse in a London teaching hospital reported the following situation:

> "There is a great inadequacy and slowness in giving adequate analgesia; in fact, it is so frequent that there is no need to give specific examples. Even when an order has been written up, nurses are slow to carry it out, even in cases where it is genuinely needed. Or the doctor does not write up analgesic for the nurses, who then have to 'bleep' him several times, while the patient is suffering much pain due to the delay."

Likewise, aged or debilitated patients may complain that nurses carelessly leave their food just out of reach, or force them to walk too quickly.[1]

---

[1] See Langslow, "Age must not invite harm or hurt", p. 20.

Much of what is complained about could well be due not to carelessness but to understaffing and other pressures which make it impossible for nurses to provide patients with all the services which they need. If so, the pressures would not always be obvious to patients, and their complaints about poor service would sometimes be unjustified. But unless these special pressures are present we have an infringement by the nurse of an ethical requirement. However, there are, once again, no intractable *moral* problems here. Any moral uncertainties which arise will centre on what a nurse should do when she witnesses another health professional infringing the requirement.

(3) Experimental treatments performed on patients

Experimentation on patients can take two forms. First, there is experimental surgery, whose effectiveness in treating a given condition is uncertain, or whose side-effects are unknown. The effectiveness or otherwise of the surgery will be ascertained only if it is performed on patients in a whole variety of conditions. Secondly, new drug treatments are being developed all the time for various conditions, and these same two questions – "How effective is it?" and "What are its side-effects?" – have to be answered, usually by means of randomized clinical trials.

The term "experimental treatments" covers many different kinds of procedure, some of them more open to moral challenge than others. Suppose that a patient has failed to respond to the more common treatments for his condition and that his physician therefore proposes some new drug treatment which, he says, might have some hope of success. Suppose also that the patient is told of the risks which the drug may involve, and, realising the desperateness of his condition, consents to the proposal. Here the doctor's action is entirely proper: he has acted throughout with the interests of his patient in mind, and has not treated him as a guinea pig for his own experimental purposes; and he has not tried to railroad him into a hasty and ill-founded decision, but has given him the information which he needs in order to decide. If the treatment in question is experimental surgery on an unconscious or in some other way incompetent patient – e.g., a young child – there could have been no question of his consenting to the procedure; but the surgeon would still have been obliged to respect him as a person, first, by explaining to his parents or guardians the options available and the risks involved; and secondly, by doing whatever he did in order to benefit the patient, not primarily in order to test the effectiveness of the experimental surgery.

Consider, on the other hand, the case of an elderly woman, Mrs. Wigley, who died in 1981 after undergoing surgery for bowel cancer. An inquest established that Mrs. Wigley had died not from the cancer itself, nor from the operation to remove it, but from bone marrow depression caused by an experimental drug which she had been given after the operation. It emerged that Mrs. Wigley had been entered in a clinical trial for this drug without her consent or even knowledge. Did those who devised and carried out this drug trial act rightly? Certainly not, if we are to go by the widespread public outrage which greeted the news of this incident.[1] In response to criticism, one of the ethical committees which had approved the clinical trial attempted to justify it on the grounds that a patient who consents to surgery thereby implicitly consents also to the drug treatments associated with the surgery, even if they are experimental. But this is disputable: the assumption of consent is reasonable only in the case of a drug treatment which is standardly used and known to be effective; it is not at all reasonable in the case of a new drug which one knows could be less beneficial than the standard one, or could have harmful side-effects. If Mrs. Wigley had been offered a choice between the two drugs – one of them standard and effective, the other experimental, with possibly beneficial but also possibly harmful effects – is it likely that she would have chosen the latter? If not, her doctors certainly would not have been justified in using it.

The usual procedure in randomized clinical trials is that the patients needing treatment for a certain condition are divided into two, or perhaps three, groups. One group are given the experimental drug being tested, while another group will be given either the standardly-used drug or a placebo; or, alternatively, we may have one group given the new drug, one given the standard prescription and a third group given a placebo. This procedure may be the only effective way of determining what advantages, if any, the new drug has over the existing one, or over the provision of no treatment at all. A trial of this sort may be justified if those taking part in it have been informed of its general nature and have accepted at least the possibility that they will be given an experimental drug or a placebo. But what if they have not been told? Is it right that they

---

[1] See the discussion of this case in M. Phillips and J. Dawson, *Doctors' Dilemmas* (Brighton, 1985), pp. 63–74.

should be entered in a clinical trail without their consent, or kept in ignorance of the fact that (e.g.) a placebo may be given?

Clearly the answer is No. Given that every human person is worthy of respect as an end in himself, it is wrong to use him as a mere means to any end, however good. He is not, then, to be coerced into participating in some research programme, or led to participate in it through being kept in ignorance of its true nature. He is to decide himself whether or not to take part. At times a refusal to participate will naturally be thought unreasonable by health professionals, as in the following example, in which we have a married couple asked to give proxy consent on behalf of their child:

> Alan Jones was admitted for routine minor surgery. He met the criteria for a randomised control trial which was being carried out at the hospital. The trial had nothing to do with Alan's condition, but researchers simply required a control group. The trial was coming to an end and only a few more cases were required. Although Alan's involvement would have entailed no more than measuring his skull and weighing him, his parents refused to allow him to be used in the research. The staff felt that they were being unnecessarily difficult and found it hard to restrain themselves from being over-persuasive.[1]

While one can understand the nurses' exasperation at the parents' apparently unreasonable attitude, the fact remains that it is up to them to decide whether their child will participate in the hospital tests or not.

Against this insistence on the necessity of gaining patients' consent for experimental treatments, it may be urged that people have a moral obligation to assist in drug trials and other experimental procedures, and hence that health professionals act rightly in involving them in such procedures without bothering to seek their consent, as in the case of Mrs. Wigley. The argument would be that established surgical and drug treatments have generally become established only because their effectiveness has been tested in clinical trials – as, for instance, in the case of vaccines for smallpox and poliomyelitis. Since we all benefit from the fact that clinical trials have been conducted in the past, we are bound, both in gratitude to those who have secured these benefits for us, and for the sake

---

[1] This case is considered by K. Melia in her article "Acts of Faith", in *Nursing Times*, vol. 84, no. 19, 11 May, 1988.

of future generations, to take part in such trials today. However, even if people are (sometimes, at least) morally obliged to take part in clinical trials, it does not follow that health professionals can enter them for such trials without their permission. It will still be up to the individual patient himself to say whether or not he wishes to be involved; he may act wrongly by refusing, but the decision is his, not some doctor's or nurse's.

Consideration of the case of Mrs. Wigley leads one to suspect that *some* doctors and nurses may be tempted to regard elderly or terminally-ill patients, and especially those who are incompetent, as "fair game" for experimental procedures. These are patients who are unable to consent to treatment, and since (as someone might argue) they are soon going to be dead whatever happens, it "does not matter" whether or not the treatment is effective or whether it produces disfiguring or painful side-effects or hastens degeneration and death. Clearly this way of treating a patient amounts to refusing to recognize his dignity as a human being. It involves viewing the patient not as an end in himself, but as a means to the benefit of other people. That this attitude is seriously wrong was pointed out by Pope Pius XII. The Pope declared that one may never deliberately sacrifice an individual person's life or physical well-being for the good of society as a whole. So, he said, it would be immoral to subject a patient to harmful experimental treatment which was not genuinely indicated as required for his own well-being; no-one may subordinate the patient as an individual to the interests of society as a whole, because "in his personal being, man is not finally ordered to usefulness to society. On the contrary, the community exists for man."[1] Likewise, the World Medical Association's Declaration of Helsinki states:

> Every biomedical research project involving human subjects should be preceded by careful assessment of predictable risks in comparison with foreseeable benefits to the subject or to others. Concern for the interests of the subject must always prevail over the interest of science and society.[2]

---

[1] Pope Pius XII, "The Moral Law and Medical Research" (an address to the First International Congress on the Histopathology of the Nervous System, 14 September, 1952). "Finally ordered" means "ordered as to an end" or "essentially orientated". To say that man is "finally ordered to usefulness in society" would be to say that every individual man finds his whole point and significance in his contribution to the good of society, the latter alone possessing a point or significance in itself and not in terms of anything further. This, of course, the Pope denies.

[2] The Declaration of Helsinki (1964; revised 1975), "Recommendations Guiding Medical Doctors in Biomedical Research Involving Human Subjects", I, para. 5

From the brief discussion in this section, and relying on the general moral principles defended in Chapters Five and Six, it is possible to set out some moral criteria which can help us to decide whether a given programme of experimental treatment is morally right. These seem to be as follows.

First, if the treatment is genuinely for the good of the patient – if it is what is called "therapeutic experimentation" – there can be no objection to it, provided that it is not in some other way intrinsically objectionable.

Secondly, if the treatment is not primarily for the patient's own good but is being pursued in order to advance human knowledge (if, that is, it is non-therapeutic experimentation) it will be more difficult to justify. The following conditions will have to be satisfied:

(i) The subject of experimentation must be informed of the general nature of the experimentation, as well as its possible risks, and must consent to take part in it. If the programme involves the use of control groups whose members are to receive placebos, the patient must be told that he *may* be placed in this group.

(ii) Since, in general, it is morally permissible for people, in a good cause, to accept certain risks to their own life and health in order to benefit others, it *may* be permissible to run such risks in a programme of experimentation. But this will be so only if the goal being aimed at is sufficiently valuable to justify accepting these risks. And, once again, the subject must be made aware of these risks and must consent to them.

(iii) On the other hand, any deliberate mutilation or injury to a subject in the interests of a research programme would be morally wrong, even if the subject were to consent to it. The reason for this conclusion is that given by Pius XII: each individual human being is an end in himself and does not have his whole point or purpose in the community of which he forms part. Hence he cannot be used as a means for benefiting the community as a whole. To accept deliberate harm for the sake of future generations (say) would amount to doing evil that good may come.

(iv) The need for informed consent seems to rule out entirely any non-therapeutic experiments involving even minor risks on children and other incompetent subjects. Consent of parents or guardians is not sufficient here: because the experimental treatment is not in the interests of the subject himself, the parents or guardians cannot reasonably presume that the subject *would* consent to undergo it if he were in a position to do so.[1]

In view of the stringent conditions which should govern the use of experimental treatments, as well as the grave injustice to patients which is likely to be involved in any immoral research programme, it is hard to see how any material co-operation by nurses in these programmes could be justified. Perhaps there could be cases of very "remote" co-operation which could be justified in certain extreme circumstances, but normally a nurse would be obliged not to take part in any experimental treatment which infringed patients' rights to be respected as persons. The kinds of research programme in which a nurse may be asked to participate are so enormously varied that a consideration of specific cases would be of little value here. The important thing is for a nurse to be aware of the moral *principles* which need to be applied to particular cases, and above all the overriding principle that the patient is always a person who is to be respected as an end in himself.

(4) Obtaining patients' consent for treatment

This requirement is a clear implication of the need to treat patients as persons, that is, as autonomous rational beings. For each patient has the ultimate responsibility for taking care of his health, and health professional are there to assist him in this task but not to take it over from him. It is, then, up to the individual patient to decide whether or not to undergo a given treatment. Doctors, nurses and others can inform and advise him, and may also attempt to persuade him to opt for one course of action rather than another, but they cannot make the decision for him. It would, then, be wrong for doctors or nurses to adopt a generally *paternalistic* attitude towards patients, that is, to do whatever they considered conducive to patients' well-being regardless of whether or not the patients wanted it or even knew what was being done. Since patients cannot help wanting to have their health maintained or restored, they can usually be expected to agree to recommendations from a health professional which

---

[1].   For a fuller treatment of the issues involved here, see B. Ashley and K. O'Rourke, *Health Care Ethics: A Theological Analysis*, section 9.4, pp. 243–251.

they believe to be in their interests. But it cannot be assumed that this is always the case, or that a patient would necessarily be acting unreasonably in rejecting a recommended treatment. There will admittedly be many situations in which one must take for granted a patient's consent to being treated and get down to work without further ado, as when a victim of a motor accident is wheeled unconscious into the operating theatre. But normally the patient must be given the information needed for deciding whether or not to agree to a proposed treatment, and then his decision must be accepted. If a patient is incompetent, the decision will have to be made by his parents or guardian, and only if they choose a course of action which is manifestly opposed to the patient's interests is there a reason for the hospital authorities to seek a court order enabling them to go ahead with a proposed treatment.

Sometimes a surgeon, while performing an operation, discovers some additional problem calling for surgery which he can rectify there and then. Would it be right to carry out this second operation, or must he complete the scheduled operation and try afterwards to obtain the patient's consent for the additional surgery? A further operation would be burdensome and to some degree dangerous for the patient; so if it is morally permissible for the surgeon to proceed directly to the second operation he should do so. He could argue that the patient's consent can reasonably be presumed, because if he were to be asked to agree to the second operation performed he would unhesitatingly do so. However, it may sometimes be doubtful whether this assumption of presumed consent is reasonable, and then a real problem of co-operation will arise for nurses in the operating theatre. The following state of affairs illustrates this problem:

A Catholic nurse working in a remote rural area in a developing country was the only person qualified to assist the medical officer in the operating theatre. A patient was admitted in obstructed labour. It seemed probable that she would never be able to deliver a child normally because of pelvic malformation, so the doctor decided to sterilize her during the caesarian section. This decision was reached without discussion with either the patient, who was physically and emotionally exhausted, or with her relatives. The nurse assisted at the operation without protest since delay could have jeopardized the patient's life. The baby was stillborn but the mother made a slow recovery. The nurse was concerned about her apparent abandonment of her moral principles and was worried about the action she should take in similar situations in the future.

Did the doctor act wrongly in sterilizing the patient? It is arguable that he did, since the procedure itself was wrong in principle, being a contraceptive and not a therapeutic sterilization: its whole point was to prevent the patient from ever again having children. (More will be said on this topic in Chapter Thirteen.) Moreover, even if the procedure itself had been free from moral objection, the doctor could not reasonably have assumed the patient's consent to it. His judgment that she would want no more children was perhaps reasonable, given her ability to give birth normally and the lack of facilities to deal with difficult births in her area. Nevertheless, the woman might have wanted to try for another another child and accept the risks involved. The doctor's action therefore amounted to treating his patient in an unjustifiably paternalistic way.

The problem for the nurse was one of co-operation. Should she have assisted the surgeon, or should she have challenged him, and perhaps refused to take any further part in the procedure, as soon as she realized what he was about to do? Or should she, out of concern for the patient's well-being, have continued assisting the surgeon during the operation but protested to him afterwards? If the sterilization itself was wrong, the second option seems clearly indicated by the principles governing co-operation in evil acts. The nurse would have acted wrongly in doing anything specifically geared to facilitating the sterilization. However, the various surgical procedures might not have been sufficiently clearly separated to enable the nurse to decide which particular acts of hers would contribute to the sterilization, and in this case, given the urgent need save the patient's life, she would evidently act rightly in continuing to assist the surgeon.

This sort of situation – a surgeon's performing surgery additional to that to which his patient has consented – may be not only immoral but unlawful as well. Under English law the doctor in the case just considered would commit an offence, and the patient would be entitled to sue him. Anyone who touches or handles a person's body without that person's consent commits the wrong or tort of battery against him or her. The consent required need not be explicitly given, but it must be reasonably presupposed. Normally, a patient who undergoes surgery in a hospital has first to fill out and sign a "Consent for Operation" form, in which he agrees to undergo the surgery in question, together with "such further or alternative operative measures as may be found necessary". Would this last phrase authorize a surgeon in acting as the doctor in the above example did? No, because the key word "necessary" has to be interpreted in a strict sense. As one legal writer explains, "The doctor is only authorized to carry out further surgery without which the patient's life or health will be immediately at risk. So the doctor discovering advanced cancer of the womb while performing a curettage may be justified in performing an immediate hysterectomy. Delay might threaten the woman's life. A doctor discovering some malformation, or other non-life-threatening condition, must delay further surgery until his patient has the opportunity to offer his opinion."[1] The same author mentions a couple of cases in which a surgeon's failure to observe these conditions hs led to his being sued for causing a battery:

> A doctor who discovered that his patient's womb was ruptured while performing minor gynaecological surgery was held liable to her for going ahead and sterilizing her there and then. She had not agreed to sterilization. A woman who underwent a hysterectomy when all she had agreed to was curettage similarly recovered for battery. The essence of the wrong of battery is the unpermitted contact.[2]

If a surgeon were to act in this way, a nurse would not be justified in co-operating with him unless a sudden withdrawal of co-operation would endanger the patient's life.

(5) Keeping patients informed

Because health professionals should avoid treating their patients paternalistically, they should never attempt either to proceed with treatment without gaining the patients' consent, or to keep them in the dark about how their cases are progressing. Patients have a definite "right to know". But just how far does this right extend? There must be some limit to it, for a doctor or nurse has no obligation to fill the patient's mind with bits of information which are of no interest or use to him. Evidently there is a minimum amount of information which the doctor is normally obliged

---

[1] M. Brazier, *Medicine, Patients and the Law* (Harmondsworth, 1987), pp. 57–58.
[2] Brazier, pp. 55–56.

to convey, the extent of this information varying from case to case, depending on the patient's condition and personal circumstances. It will always include any information which, if known to the patient, could reasonably be expected to influence him either for or against treatment. For it is up to him to decide whether or not to proceed with treatment, and to make this decision he needs to be given all the relevant information. The point of contemporary talk about *informed* consent" to treatment is that respect for patients as persons requires that they be provided with that knowledge – of their conditions, and of the nature and effects of the treatment proposed – which they need in order to decide whether to consent or not. A doctor who withholds information because he fears that only in this way can he obtain his patient's consent acts wrongly. He cannot, then, expect nurses to co-operate with him in keeping the information hidden from the patient. Nurses have, in fact, every right to refuse to collaborate in such attempts to hide vital information.

(6) Respecting patients' beliefs and cultural background

The Code of Ethics issued by CICIAMS in 1972 states that the nurse is obliged to provide the services which her patients need regardless of who those patients are and what moral and religious beliefs they hold:

> The nurse cares for patients conscientiously and with an equal devotion whatever the race, nationality, social class, political opinions, philosophical convictions or religious beliefs of those committed to his or her care. He or she respects everyone's legitimate freedom of conscience.[1]

However, the code does not explain the difference between legitimate and illegitimate freedom of conscience, nor does it indicate how a nurse should respond when, by accommodating herself to a patient's moral or religious beliefs (or the lack of them), she would act against her own conscience. We may, for instance, have a patient exerting pressure on a nurse to do something for him which the nurse considers immoral; or, conversely, we may have a patient making what the nurse considers an immoral refusal of treatment. In the first situation the nurse may not do something which is morally wrong; the fact that she is urged to do it by a

---

[1] CICIAMS, *Code of Ethics* (1972), p. 4 ("Fundamental Moral Values", no. 4).

patient is irrelevant. In both cases, moreover, she may find it difficult not to disagree openly with the patient; but whether or not she should express disagreement will depend on several factors, including that of how receptive he would be to her comments.

How should health professionals react when the parent or guardian of an incompetent patient refuses permission, on moral grounds, for an operation which is necessary to save the patient's life? An obvious example here is that of a Jehovah's Witness parent who refuses to countenance a blood transfusion for his child even though without it he will probably die. Often, in such cases, hospitals have obtained court orders taking the matter out of the parents' hands; and in cases of emergency, medical teams may go ahead and give the transfusion, thus disregarding the parent's instruction, and to leave the legal problems to be sorted out after the child's life has been saved. (Fortunately, situations of this kind do not occur as frequently as they used to, because surgical teams are becoming more and more adept at doing away with the need for blood transfusions; but they do still occur.) It could be argued that because the parent has rightful authority over his child, an authority which is delegated to the hospital team at certain times of need but is not wholly transferred to them, the hospital authorities should not attempt to override this authority even when they believe that it is being used wrongly. On this view, while the Jehovah's Witness parents may be objectively mistaken in holding blood transfusions to be immoral, given that they do sincerely hold this belief, we should not prevent them from acting in accordance with it. But it is also arguable that to deprive a child of life-saving treatment is so radical an injustice that it would be wrong not to intervene and give the transfusion. On this view the parents can be seen as hostile to the interests of their child, and their wishes in his regard may therefore be overridden – just as a child can be made a ward of court if his parents are grossly mistreating him.

The argument against allowing the child's parents to prohibit a life-saving transfusion seems particularly strong. For although parents do have authority over their children, this authority is not absolute but has definite limits. The child is himself an individual person and not the property of his parents, and if the parents propose something which manifestly threatens grave injury to his life and health, other people, including health professionals, are not obliged to sit around and allow them to carry out that proposal. So, "the child has a basic right to life and health; accordingly, the parents may not compromise that right but are obliged to promote it. Since the child is not yet capable of assenting freely to the religious belief regarding blood transfusions, the parents speak for the child. But their decision-making should be for the *best interests of the child*. The *child's* conscience would *not* be violated if "forced" to accept a life-saving transfusion."[1] Certainly the nurse who is appalled by the harm which threatens the child as a result of his parent's refusal of life-preserving treatment could hardly be said to act wrongly by taking part in the provision of blood for the patient against his parent's wishes.

(7) *Respecting the unconscious or otherwise incompetent patient*

There are two main reasons why it is worthwhile to focus explicitly on incompetent patients. First, if a patient is incompetent he will be unable to recognise or complain about the fact that he is not being treated with the same care that a competent patient would receive; so there may be a temptation for health professionals to treat some incompetent patients in an unacceptable mannner. Secondly, some medical researchers may regard certain groups of incompetent patients as "fair game" for surgical and pharmacological experimentation. And their attitude would be supported by those contemporary philosophers who argue that human beings who lack such crucial abilities as the power to think coherently and reason, and to form an intelligible conception of themselves as individual entities, are not persons and hence do not deserve to be treated as persons.[2] This philosophical issue is central here. Does (say) a comatose patient qualify as a human person, or is he (as such expressions as "persistent vegetative state" suggest) now existing at a sub-personal level? If comatose people (and human embryos, newborn infants, the

---

[1]. "Jehovah's Witnesses and Blood", in *Ethics & Medics*, May 1982. This article insists, however, that even for one who rejects the Jehovah's Witnesses' moral convictions concerning blood transfusions, "it is vital that respect for their conscience be strictly maintained by health care personnel so long as a basic right of a third party is not seriously violated." The author appeals here to the Second Vatican Council's Declaration on Religious Liberty, which states that ". . . all men should be immune from coercion on the part of individuals, social groups and every human power so that, within due limits, nobody is forced to act against his convictions in religious matters in private or public, alone or in association with others."

[2]. A clearly expressed and apparently influential exposition of this argument, which is taken to justify even infanticide in certain cases, appears in Michael Tooley's *Abortion and Infanticide* (Oxford, 1983). See also Helga Kuhse and Peter Singer, *Should the Baby Live?* (Oxford, 1985) pp. 131–3.

terminally-ill, etc.) are not human persons, then presumably we need feel no more qualms about experimenting on them than on monkeys or rats. This whole question will be taken up in Chapter Thirteen, concerning abortion. To anticipate some results of that discussion here, I suggest that one may describe the condition of comatose people in a way which parallels that of the human embryo and foetus. A three-month-old foetus is a human being in the full sense, a person, but one whose natural capacities and potentialities are at present in a radically undeveloped state: it is an *immature* specimen of humanity. Likewise, someone in a comatose state is still a human person, but one whose characteristically human capacities and potentialities cannot be expressed in normal mental and physical activity because of damage to his brain. The brain damage is an impediment to the utilization of the patient's mental and physical capacities, but the capacities themselves, and therefore the human nature of which they are characteristic, continue to exist in him. Hence there is no justification for treating a comatose patient as a non-person. The fact that he is comatose may well justify us in rejecting certain forms of life-preserving treatment as pointless; but this is a far cry from the conclusion endorsed by some recent "quality-of-life" theorists, that in dealing with a comatose patient we can dispense with the "niceties" which we have to observe in treating competent human beings.

(8) Caring for mentally-ill patients

An entire book could be devoted to ethical problems raised by nursing care for mentally-ill patients; here I shall consider only a few of the most pressing of such problems.

The words "mental illness" apply to a wide range of conditions, from neurotic conditions which do not call for hospitalization to severe psychoses such as schizophrenia and criminal insanity which require patients to be confined to a secure environment where they can undergo psychiatric treatment. And mental hospitals typically house not only the mentally ill but also the grossly mentally retarded, those who cannot hope to live outside special institutions. Because patients in mental hospitals cannot deal, intellectually or emotionally, with many problems of day-to-day living and may, in some cases, be unable to speak coherently or to take note of what is going on around them, they will often be unaware that they are not being treated with the respect due to them – that, for instance, proper nursing care is not being provided. Because of this, the temptation for a health professional to neglect the proper care of these patients may be greater than in the case of patients who are mentally normal. This temptation will be accentuated if a patient is manifestly irrational or offensive or violent. In such a case, the easiest way of handling him may be to put him in solitary confinement for long stretches of the day. It may also be thought necessary to use force to administer some tranquillizing drugs. Both these types of action may sometimes be legitimate, but equally are open to abuse. If a patient is behaving in a violent and dangerous way and is impervious to all reasonable appeals for calm, it may indeed be necessary to sedate him forcibly; and sometimes the best way of dealing with a troublesome patient – best for himself and also for everyone else in the institution – may be to place him in seclusion. On the other hand, there certainly are cases in which seclusion is resorted to for the wrong reasons. The report *Conscientious Objectors at Work*, published some years ago by the investigative group Social Audit, mentions several such cases. According to this report, some nurses interviewed during the investigation were concerned about "the possibility that patients were secluded unnecessarily, or deprived of their rights under the Mental Health Act 1959". The report included the following statements by two mental nurses:

> "Unauthorised seclusion was used to keep hyperactive residents out of the way during the day. . ."

> ". . . a patient with Huntington's Chorea was often in seclusion while staff had hour-long breakfast/lunch/tea breaks, as she was considered a nuisance."[1]

The same report contains the following record of an evidently improper use of tranquillizing drugs:

> "A forty-three year old severely subnormal woman (ambulant) was placed on a ward for physically handicapped patients who sit round in chairs for most of the day. She had a habit of grabbing people for attention and had quite a firm grip. She was also noisy. . . Often she would be sat in a chair and the tray tightened so that she could not move it, to keep her out of the way of staff. Eventually staff complained about her grabbing and noise, so for lack of a more

---

1. V. Beardshaw, *Conscientious Objectors at Work* (London, 1981), p. 19.

suitable ward she was placed on a more secure ward and her medication – chlorpromazine – increased to keep her quiet. She is often defenceless against violent and aggressive attacks from other patients".[1]

Given the obstructive and irritating behaviour displayed by this woman, it is understandable that the staff were tempted to treat her as they did. They nevertheless acted wrongly, because although it may have been in the patient's interest to have her medication increased, when the staff had her consigned to a ward where she was be in danger of attack from other patients they were promoting only their own convenience.

While inconsiderate and cruel treatment of patients cannot be justified, it is sometimes (as in the case just considered) easy to understand how nurses could act in this way. For mentally-ill patients are often particularly difficult to handle precisely because their personalities are disordered, and they are often highly vulnerable because they are unaware of the way in which they should be treated and cannot complain if it turns out that they are treated badly. In addition, the public funding of mental hospitals in Britain is notoriously inadequate, and such institutions are often badly maintained and equipped, with shortages of staff or with staff who are unsuited to work in such an environment. In these circumstances it is hardly surprising if the ethos and morale of mental hospitals is not always what it should be, and that abuses do occur.

Three ethical problems are particularly important here: first, the use of force on violent patients; secondly, the administration of drugs; and thirdly, the administration of electro-convulsive therapy. Are these practices morally licit? If so, when, under what circumstances?

(i) *The use of force on violent patients.* Problems to do with the use of force are by no means confined to mental nursing, for nurses and doctors may forcibly restrain non-mentally-ill patients, or compel them to submit to a given form of treatment. Where this happens to a patient who is capable of making his own decisions about medical treatment, there is a morally wrong use of force, because the choice of the patient as a rational and free agent is being overridden. What, however, if the patient, due to mental illness or mental handicap, cannot reach conclusions about the advisability or otherwise of treatment in a rational way?

---

[1] *ibid.*

Consider another type of situation in which health professionals proceed with treatment without first gaining the patient's consent. A man has been badly injured in a car accident; he is brought unconscious into a hospital, and the surgical team sets to work straight away to try to save his life. What justifies them in operating without having gained the patient's consent? The answer, evidently, is that the patient was at the time *incapable* of consenting to the operation, but that since it was manifestly in his interest to undergo it, he would have consented if he had been able to consider the matter. Hence his consent can be reasonably presumed. The same principle would justify a surgical team in operating on a small child after the child's parents had consented, even though he had protested that he did not want to go into hospital. It would be argued that the child is too immature to appreciate what is involved in the operation, or the grave consequences of not undergoing it, and therefore that despite his opposition to going into hospital, he could be deemed to have implicitly consented to the procedure. The same principles apply in the case of mentally-ill patients. If a patient is incapable of making a rationally-founded decision to accept a proposed treatment, and if the treatment is manifestly in his interests, one may impose the treatment on him even if, in so doing, coercion has to be used. For it can be reasonably presumed that if the patient were able to think about the matter coolly and rationally he would give his consent. But the two conditions placed on this use of the notion of "reasonable presumption" must be kept in mind here: first, the proposed treatment must benefit the patient, and secondly, the patient himself must be incapable of thinking in a rational manner about it. If the patient's aversion to treatment is to be overridden, it must be on the grounds that emotional or other non-rational factors have prevented him from reasoning coherently and consistently about the matter. Clearly this will apply to some but by no means all mentally-ill patients: there can be no question of giving *carte blanche* for doctors and nurses to coerce mentally-ill patients into undergoing treatment.

(ii) *The administration of drugs.* The drugs with which we are concerned here are the psychotropic drugs, which, by acting chemically on the brain, can alter a patient's mood and behaviour. There are now many such drugs, ranging from the relatively mild – sleeping tablets, tranquillizers such as Valium, and anti-depressants – to the so-called major tranquillizers or antipsychotic drugs such as chlorpromazine and thioradizine. Most of the ethical problems involved in administering drugs concern this last group. The following description of their common effects on patients will make it clear why this should be so.

Antipsychotic drugs have a wide range of clinical uses:

1. They exert a quietening effect on severely disturbed patients.

2. They diminish certain special features of psychotic illness such as hallucinations and delusions. They are the main treatment of schizophrenia, especially in its acute form.

3. They prevent or postpone relapses in chronic schizophrenic illnesses.

[The action of these drugs] ... is primarily to combat symptoms rather than to alter the mechanism underlying a particular condition. Used as major tranquillizers, they are often administered to very disturbed patients who are hostile, aggressive and otherwise uncontrollable...

The side-effects of antipsychotic drugs severely limit their usefulness. Common among them are dry mouth, blurred vision, constipation, dizziness, falls in blood pressure and a pounding heart... [V]oluntary movement becomes increasingly difficult; the patient's expression becomes fixed and mask-like... his hands tremble... In other patients the drug may induce painful muscular spasms or severe restlessness. Happily all these effects disappear when the drug is discontinued or the dosage lowered.

A much more worrying side-effect is the condition known as tardive diskinesia, characterised by repetitive involuntary movements of a tremulous, twitching or writhing nature involving the mouth, lips, tongue, trunk and limbs. In mild degrees it is unsightly and upsetting. In more severe degrees it interferes with eating and breathing. The condition is sometimes irreversible.[1]

Given that the effects of these drugs are so severe, it would be right to administer them only if the patient's condition is so serious that it justifies one in accepting these effects on him. It would be wrong to use them on a

---

[1]. Council for Science and Society, *Treating the Troublesome: The ethical problems of compulsory medical treatment for socially unacceptable behaviour; The report of a working party* (London, 1981), p. 7.

patient just because he was demanding of one's attention or annoying to other patients. Only if he were violent or aggressively offensive would one be justified in using them to control his behaviour – and then, since this behaviour would be harmful for the patient himself, the drugs would work for his own benefit as well as for that of others.

The first ethical constraint on the use of these drugs is, then, that they may be used only when the condition of the patient is of such gravity as to require them; the treatment must, in other words, be proportionate to the condition for which it is prescribed. A second constraint can be derived from some observations of Pope Pius XII, which apply generally to the treatment of all kinds of conditions.[1] The Pope pointed out that man, as a being with rational as well as emotional and sensory powers, needs to respect the natural hierarchy which obtains between these powers. His emotional and sensory functions should be governed by reason, and in acting he should decide rationally and freely what to do. While, then, it is legitimate to use surgery, drugs or other techniques to combat pain or suffering or anti-social behaviour, it would be wrong to do so if this involved a constant and more or less long-term loss of the patient's ability to deliberate and decide on his actions. Hence, antipsychotic drugs may not be administered to a patient if they are so powerful that whatever ability he has to think and choose rationally will be taken away from him. If he would be deprived of this ability, but intermittently rather than constantly, such drugs could still be used. But if the patient were to be more or less permanently deprived of his rational abilities, it would be immoral to administer them. On the other hand, it may be that the patient's psychotic condition is itself so severe as to eliminate any possibility of his thinking rationally and deciding freely, in which case the administration of drugs would not really take anything valuable away from him. The problems which arise here are admittedly difficult, and, like many other problems in bioethics, cannot be handled by any simple application of hard-and-fast rules. But the two principles outlined here – concerning the proportionality of treatment to the patient's condition, and concerning respect for the natural hierarchy of powers in the human person – need always to be borne in mind.

---

[1]   Pius XII's teaching is contained in his Allocution to the First International Congress of Histopathology on September 14, 1952. A valuable recent discussion of this teaching is B. M. Ashley and K. D. O'Rourke, *Health Care Ethics: A Theological Analysis* (St. Louis, U.S.A., 1981, pp. 351–353.

(iii) *The administration of electro-convulsive therapy.* What happens when a patient undergoes electro-convulsive therapy (ECT) is that an electric current is passed briefly through his brain, inducing an epileptic fit. The way in which this procedure works is as yet only imperfectly understood, but it can greatly benefit some patients suffering from severe depression. Of these patients, it is claimed, three quarters or even more recover completely after a course of several administrations of ECT, spread over a period of three to four weeks. Some forms of schizophrenia also apparently respond well to this treatment.[1] ECT delivers such a severe shock to the central nervous system that physiological states which underlie conditions such as depression can be altered quite radically, with the result that the conditions themselves may disappear.

The principal ethical question arising here would seem to be: Is this shock to the system so radical as to be morally objectionable? Is it disproportionate to the benefits foreseen from it? The answer, evidently, is "No". First, the benefits to be gained by the use of ECT – elimination of severe depression and amelioration of certain types of schizophrenia – are immensely valuable for the patient himself. Secondly, although ECT does involve disturbing a person's central nervous system in a way which would be wrong if done for trivial reasons, it does not seem to impart any injury which could outweigh the benefits regularly resulting from it. The principal adverse effect of ECT is a certain loss of memory, although this loss varies in extent from person to person and may in any case be only temporary. But this damage to one's memory is a side-effect of the treatment, and we are surely justified in tolerating it in view of the benefits likely to result for the patient. In addition, although ECT does carry some small risk to the life of the patient, this risk has to be set against the risk of suicide which is always present in someone who is severely depressed.[2] We can say, then, that although ECT can be misused, it does have legitimate uses, and that these uses are legitimate because of the genuine benefit which the technique promises to many mentally-ill people.

★　★　★

---

[1]. Cf. Council for Science and Society, *Treating the Troublesome,* pp. 8–9.
[2]. *ibid.*

This Chapter in Summary

Nurses and other health professionals have an obligation to respect patients by treating them as persons, that is, as rational beings possessing free will who are capable of deciding for themselves whether or not to undergo treatment. This obligation to respect patients as persons obviously rules out all paternalistic treatment of them: the health professional must inform the patient about his condition and what is proposed to cope with it, and he must obtain the patient's free and informed consent for treatment. Since there are many ways in which a patient may *not* be treated with respect, the title of the chapter, "Treating Patients with Respect", covers a wide range of duties towards patients. Relying on the principle of respect for persons, we can set out criteria for deciding whether or not a given programme of experimental treatment is morally acceptable. It is clear that some programmes of experimentation on human subjects are immoral in themselves and that nurses should not co-operate in them. Some especially difficult problems arise when we consider problems concerning mentally-ill patients, for whom there may be no possibility of giving free and informed consent to treatment: problems concerning the use of force, the administration of psychotropic drugs and recourse to electro-convulsive therapy deserve consideration here. It is concluded that all three may be morally justified, but only under strictly limited conditions.

CHAPTER NINE

PROBLEMS OF HONESTY AND CONFIDENTIALITY

The problems which now need to be discussed typically concern the issue of whether one should tell the truth rather than lie, and the related issue of whether one is obliged to tell the whole truth or may instead disclose only part of the information which one possesses. These problems are encountered by people in all walks of life, but they seem to arise with particular frequency and urgency in the health-care field.

Concerning specifically those issues of honesty and confidentiality which affect nursing practice, a common problem is that of whether a nurse should sometimes, or even always, disclose to a patient details of his prognosis or course of treatment which his doctor (or, perhaps, his family) wants withheld from him. Secondly, problems may often arise because nurses are unsure how much the patient (or his family) has already been told, and are therefore undecided what to say to the patient in their ordinary dealings with him. Thirdly, a patient may give a nurse information which he insists is to be kept confidential, and if this information has some bearing on his treatment the nurse will have to ask herself whether she should share it with her professional colleagues, thereby breaking the undertaking she has given. Fourthly, we have problems which arise because patients are sometimes not presented with the facts on which to make a judgment for or against treatment. Since it is normally assumed that the patient has the right to know these facts, any attempt to conceal them from him is regarded as an attempt at deliberate deception. Finally, there are problems involved in administering placebos. Let us look briefly at these issues one by one.

(1) Giving the patient information which one has been told to keep from him

Consider the following incident, which was reported by a nurse at a London hospital:

"When a patient asked me if she would ever leave the hospital alive there was no way I could tell her to ask the Sister, as the patient had

163

specifically said: 'I want to ask *you*, and I know that you wouldn't lie to me.' At the time I told her that we were doing all we could and that she could help too, by co-operating fully with her treatment, so that she could eventually walk out of hospital. But I hate fobbing people off with answers like that, because I know that I would resent someone's doing that to me. And I believe that if a person wants to know the truth and is capable of handling it emotionally it is unfair of us to keep it from him. It is his right to know."

This report raises three closely-related problems. First, would it be right to lie to the patient? A nurse must face this question, because unless she has resolved to answer the patient's questions truthfully, regardless of the doctor's instruction, she will be strongly tempted to tell a lie. Should she yield to the temptation or not? The nurse who reported this incident considered it wrong to lie, and tried to satisfy the patient with an evasive answer. Secondly, this nurse and her patient have evidently built up a close personal relationship, as is shown by the patient's trust in the nurse. This relationship of respect and trust is in itself an immensely valuable thing which would be imperilled if she were to lie to the patient, even though the damage would not be done until the patient became aware of the deception. But would not the nurse also damage this relationship by answering the patient's questions evasively? For if patients realize that their questions are being evaded, they may become disillusioned with their nurses as people on whose honesty they can rely. Finally, does a patient normally have a strict right to be told the details of his diagnosis, his course of treatment and his prospects? If he does, then his doctor should tell him what he wants to know about these things and may neither withhold the information from him nor direct nurses to withhold it. A nurse may then be morally entitled to go against the doctor's instructions and tell the patient what he wants to know. Would she have been entitled to do this in the situation described above?

The crucial question

If we are to resolve the problems presented by this nurse's report we must tackle the central moral issue which it raises. Is it wrong to tell a lie? Is lying wrong only in general, so that on some occasions it would be morally acceptable to lie, or is it an intrinsically wrong activity which cannot be justified under any circumstances? And if we answer "Yes" to the second question, can we nevertheless add that some other forms of deception are sometimes morally licit? As it happens, these questions have been much debated over the years by Catholic moral theologians; indeed, they have probably been considered much more carefully and deeply in Catholic circles than in any others. In trying to identify what exactly is wrong with lying I shall draw heavily on this Catholic tradition.

Is it wrong to tell a lie? A utilitarian thinker would have to say that there is nothing wrong with lying in itself, and that it will be wrong only when it fails to produce the best possible consequences; but when lying would produce better consequences than would telling the truth, it would be not only permissible but obligatory to lie. In support of his claim, the utilitarian could adduce various "extreme situations" in which, apparently, the only way to avoid terrible harm is to lie. For instance: A gang of armed men enter the office of the local newspaper and order the secretary to show them into the editor's office. The secretary knows that the editor has made powerful enemies through his fearless exposure of local businessmen's involvement in drug trafficking; she realizes that the gangsters probably intend to kill him. She knows also that the editor is in his office across the corridor, sitting at his desk, a perfect target for the gunman. She decides that if she says to the gunman "He's not here; he went out to the bank five minutes ago" she may be able to deceive them and thus save the editor's life. Would she act rightly in doing this? Many of us would answer that she would, and the utilitarian would go further. He would claim that provided the proposed response was likely to be the most effective way of throwing the gunmen off the scent, it would be not only acceptable but obligatory: the secretary would act wrongly in doing anything else.

Natural-law moralists have traditionally held that lying is wrong in principle, that no lie can ever be justified, not even a so-called "white lie". If the option which faces us is that of telling a lie or allowing some catastrophe to take place, then, they have said, we are morally obliged to suffer the catastrophe: to seek to avert it by lying would be to "do evil that good may come". They have tended to base this claim that lying is absolutely excluded on arguments focusing on what a person actually does when he tells a lie, but have also appealed to certain biblical texts which appear to be decisive: "Lie not one to another" (Colossians 3, 9); "Wherefore, put away lying and speak truth every man with his neighbour" (Ephesians 4, 25). Many protestant theologians, however, have been prepared to admit some lies as permitted or even obligatory. So we find, for example, that a contributor to a widely-used dictionary of Christian ethics has this to say:

> There is no doubt in general of the evil of lying. It destroys the basis of human association and in the end is stultifying. Christian thought, however, down the centuries has been much exercised whether it is ever right to tell a lie... In a controversy with St. Jerome, St. Augustine wrote two treatises against lies in any circumstances (*De Mendacio* and *Contra Mendacium*). Centuries later he was to be followed by the philosopher Kant... It is clear that there may be circumstances in which it is right to tell a lie, but most people tell lies when they should not. The temptation comes swiftly and they succumb. Perhaps it is to get out of an awkward situation, or to practise some petty fraud or deception. The only way to have the sensitivity of spirit to know when a lie is called for in particular circumstances is to be habitually truthful.[1]

In view of the very strong Christian tradition of rejection of all lying, this author's judgment that "it is clear that there may be circumstances in which it is right to tell a lie" is hasty, to say the least. Moreover, his concluding statement – "The only way to have the sensitivity of spirit to know when a lie is called for in particular circumstances is to be habitually truthful" – appears confused. For either "to be habitually truthful" means "to be always truthful" (or, perhaps, "to endeavour to be always truthful") or it does not. If it does, the author is contradicting himself, because he is saying that if one attempts always to be truthful one will then be able to acquire the "sensitivity of spirit" to know when not to be truthful! If on the other hand "to be habitually truthful" means only "to be truthful for the most part, or on the great majority of occasions, or whenever truthfulness is morally demanded", or something like that, it hardly seems correct to say that one's habitual truthfulness, in this sense, will give one the required "sensitivity"; for one who has built up this kind of habitual truthfulness, since he is already prepared to lie on some occasions, will already have decided when he may depart from his general rule against lying and when he may not. And we will have no grounds for thinking that his decision to make exceptions in favour of lying in such-

---

1. R. Preston, "Lying", in J. Macquarrie (ed.), *A Dictionary of Christian Ethics* (London, 1967), p. 202.

and-such circumstances was a correct decision. So this appeal to an "habitual truthfulness" which falls short of absolute truthfulness fails to establish what the author wants to establish.

While Catholic moralists, following St. Augustine and St. Thomas, have tended to agree on the basic principle that lying is in itself wrong and therefore always excluded, they have sometimes disagreed over their answers to two other questions: first, Why is it that lying is wrong – what is it about lying that makes it wrong?; and secondly, How do we determine what is a lie and what is not? This second question is particularly important, because some Catholic moralists claim that in certain extreme circumstances a statement which would normally be regarded as a lie could turn out not to be so, and hence would not be open to moral objection. They could argue, for instance, that because of the gunmen's threat of unjust violence to the newspaper editor, the secretary's reply to them does not count as a lie, even though it appears, on the surface, to be one. Let us look a little more closely at these two vital questions.

First, what is it about lying that makes it a wrong act? Various answers are given to this question. Consider, for instance, the argument contained in the article on "Lying" in the *New Catholic Encyclopaedia*, which provides a handy summary of Christian teaching and theorizing about truth-telling and lying. First of all the author defines lying as

> An act contrary to truthfulness, or the virtue of veracity, consisting in the communication to another of a judgment that is not in accord with what the one who communicates it thinks to be true.[1]

Following the usual practice, he then distinguishes between three kinds of lie. First, there is the lie which is told in jest or for the purpose of amusement (the so-called "jocose lie"[2]); secondly, there is the lie which one tells in order to achieve some useful good or to prevent some misfortune from occurring (the "officious lie"); and finally, there is the lie which is consciously intended to harm another person (the "pernicious lie"). He then produces the following argument:

> The most fundamental argument is that drawn from man's social nature. The social order that human nature requires for its proper

---

[1] D. Hughes, "Lying", *New Catholic Encyclopaedia*, Vol. 8, pp. 1107–1110, at p. 1107.

[2] This expression covers lies which are told to a person simply for the pleasure of misleading him, without being motiviated by any desire for gain or any seriously malicious intent.

development and fulfilment demands that mutual trust and confidence and a general friendly good will should prevail between men. This, however, is undermined not only by the pernicious lie that damages the rights and reputations of others, but also by officious and jocose lies, because if one were under no obligation to refrain from such lies, an individual's confidence in the communications made to him would be considerably lowered. Every statement would have to be weighed with suspicion, and this would, in effect, debase the currency of communication. Man's faculty of speech or communication would be perverted in the sense that the prevalent mendacity would make it impossible or difficult to communicate with others. This is a situation that has in fact come to pass in matters with regard to which "white" or "social" lies are in common use. Words lose their meaning and their capacity to convey thought. Richard Cabot [in his book *Honesty* (New York, 1938)] has pointed out the dilemma that physicians create for themselves when, for human reasons, they lie to patients suffering from disease. When this practice comes to be generally known, the physician has no effective way of reassuring a patient who suspects that he has contracted such and such a disease and that his physician is concealing this fact. [1]

The kernel of this argument is that "if one were under no obligation to refrain from such lies [*sc.* lies of all three kinds], an individual's confidence in communications made to him would be considerably lowered." This claim concerning the likely consequences of people's failing to observe an absolute prohibition against lying is open to some doubt. For surely what is needed to maintain "an individual's confidence in the communications made to him" is not necessarily an *absolute prohibition* of lying, but (say) a prohibition that holds good in all but extreme and hence rare circumstances. In other words, the reliability of human communication could be based solely on the general and overall truthfulness of people's statements, that is, their being true in all but quite exceptional circumstances. So this particular argument for the wrongness of lying is inconclusive. On the other hand the argument contains much of value, because it is true that the communication of knowledge, an immensely valuable aspect of human life, is put seriously at risk by the practice of lying. In other words,

---

[1.] Hughes, "Lying", p. 1107.

a large part of the point of human discourse is to *communicate the way things are*. When a person lies he acts against this prime aim of speech or discourse and uses it for an exactly contrary purpose, namely, to communicate that which is not the case. As St. Thomas Aquinas says:

> Because our statements function naturally as signs of what is in our understanding, it is unnatural and inappropriate that any statement express something which we do not, in fact, have in our minds.

What is essentially the same condemnation of lying has often been expressed in the argument that in lying the faculty of speech is abused. As one moral theologian puts it:

> Lying is the expression of thoughts that are contrary to intellectual conviction. Therefore the essence of a lie is the contradiction between the outward expression and the interior conviction. The social effect of the lie is to deceive. Its primary and essential immorality is not, however, based on the violation of the rights of others to the truth nor on the social harm that lying inflicts. A lie is intrinsically, and necessarily, by its very nature, contrary to the law of Nature and is, therefore, a morally evil act. The essence of the evil of lying consists in the abuse of the faculty of speech, for the primary purpose of speech is to reveal what is in the mind, whereas, in lying, that purpose is frustrated in the very act of speech.[2]

Now the basic human good which is at stake in communication is the good of knowledge, and knowledge is, by definition, knowledge of that which is the case, that which is true. Since someone who tells a lie severs the connexion which normally holds between human discourse and what is taken to be true, to tell a lie is as such to attack directly the basic good of knowledge in the person of one's hearer. Like a number of basic ethical arguments, this argument is the expression of a whole way of looking at some aspect of human life and can hardly be stated in a way that would convince someone who professed to see no harm in occasional lying. Given that the good of knowledge is one of the basic human goods and is therefore of immense importance to human life, there are certain ways of behaving when this good is at stake which are ruled out from the start, as

---

1. St. T. Aquinas, *Summa Theologiae*, part 2–2, question 110, article 3.
2. H. Davis, S.J., *Moral and Pastoral Theology*, Vol. II (*"Commandments of God, Precepts of the Church"*), p. 411.

incompatible with the respect which we should have for that good. One such action will be that of deliberately asserting something which one knows to be at odds with the truth, and this means that lying is wrong. Some lies will, of course, be much less gravely wrong than others, but *all* lies, whether "white" or serious, will be immoral and to be avoided in all circumstances.

What, then, do we say about one's duty in those extreme circumstances in which one is threatened with violence to give information to someone who has no right to it, as in the case of the gunmen who demand to know the whereabouts of the newspaper editor? It is arguable that those threatening violence in such cases thereby destroy the conditions under which genuine human communication or discourse may take place, so that a statement which would normally count as a lie would, *under these extreme circumstances*, not do so.[1] I am not endorsing this proposed solution here, only recording the fact that it is accepted by many people who adhere to the principle that lying is always wrong. Whether it is a correct solution or not, it is clear that the pressures on a nurse to withhold information from one of her patients concerning the patient's own condition and prospects are not of this extreme sort. For in the first place, the information in question is something to which the patient normally has a right: he is not seeking to know something which is no business of his. And secondly, even though the nurse may suffer unfortunate consequences by telling the patient the truth, these consequences do not compare in gravity with the violent attack which the gunmen intend to unleash upon the newspaper editor.

So a nurse is obliged always to tell the truth to her patients; she may not lie to them. To say this is not, however, to claim that she must always tell them the *whole* truth; if there are good reasons for her withholding part of the truth from a patient, she may do so. If, for example, it were apparent that a patient's request for information about his condition was half-hearted and that the purpose of his request was to receive as much reassurance as possible, it would certainly be legitimate for the nurse to

---

[1]   Cf. D. Hughes, "Lying", p. 1110. This solution to the problem is supported also by the moral theologian Fr. Henry Davis, S.J. After arguing that lying is as such immoral, he adds: "Now as speech is for social use, it is obvious that a lie is not possible unless one speaks in such circumstances as to be rightly thought to be speaking in a human way and to be communicating one's actual thoughs, or to be rightly appearing to do so. Thus, if one is unjustly forced to speak under undue pressure, speech is not then human; no one could think so. If the hearer thinks it is, he deceives himself." (H. Davis, S.J., *Moral and Pastoral Theology*, vol. II, p. 412.)

emphasize the positive aspects of his condition and to play down, or even to omit any mention of, the negative aspects. But if a patient makes it clear that he wants to know all the facts about his condition, the bad as well as the good, then it is wrong for doctors or nurses to withhold these facts from him.

From a Christian point of view there is an especially strong objection to keeping dying patients in the dark. For since each patient is a human person with an eternal destiny for which his life on earth is a preparation, it is vital that he be aware of his impending death so that he can make his peace with God and with other persons with whom he may need to be reconciled, and so that he can settle his temporal affairs.[1]

Suppose, then, that a doctor fails in his duty of informing a patient of the likelihood that he will die. What should be a nurse's response if she is questioned by the patient, as in the situation recorded a few pages back? One thing she must not do is support the doctor by telling the patient a lie. But must she tell the patient the truth *immediately*, in response to his question? Not necessarily; she would be justified in giving some more or less evasive response ("I really can't say", or something like that), and trying to decide, after talking over the matter with colleagues, what further action to take. The nature of this further action cannot be settled in advance, because much will depend on facts concerning this particular patient, the consultant's relations with the patient and his family, conditions among staff at the hospital, and so on. (It could be, for instance, that discussing the matter with the doctor himself would be the most effective way of resolving the situation.) But if it is clear that the patient wants to know the information which the doctor is withholding from him, he must be told, if not by the nurse herself, then perhaps by one of her more senior colleagues. This is an area in which the notion of the nurse as an independent health professional has serious implications for clinical practice. A nurse would be untrue to her professional calling and betray her professional responsibility if she were to allow herself to accede to a request for concealment of information vitally affecting the patient simply because this request came from another health professional.

---

[1] The *Code of Medical Ethics for Catholic Hospitals* adopted in 1954 by many Catholic dioceses in the United States expresses this obligation clearly: "Everyone has the right and the duty to prepare for the solemn moment of death. Unless it is clear, therefore, that a dying patient is already well-prepared for death as regards both temporal and spiritual affairs, it is the physician's duty to inform him of his critical condition or to have some other responsible person impart this information." (Quoted in G. Kelly, S.J., *Medico-Moral Problems*, p. 42.)

(2) Confusion about what the patient knows and does not know

It is typical of work in the health professions that individual patients will each be the responsibility of not one but several people over a short period of time – different hospital consultants, nurses on different shifts, social workers, etc. This can lead to situations in which it is uncertain what has been said to the patient about his condition, and how much the various other health professionals know about his case. Consider the following state of affairs:

> A patient was apparently ignorant of the fact that he was terminally ill. As far as was known he had not availed himself of opportunities to question the medical and nursing staff about his prognosis and it was impossible to know whether he was aware of the situation but preferred not to discuss it or whether he really was ignorant of his prognosis. He was discharged from hospital under the care of the community terminal care team. Since he had no family to provide support, the community nurse wanted to mobilize immediate help from the social services, but the best way of obtaining swift action was to explain the nature and severity of the patient's illness. This concerned the nurse, since it would entail giving confidential information to people outside the health care team without the possibility of obtaining the patient's consent.

This situation poses two distinct problems, one purely factual and the other moral. The factual problem is that there is no apparent way of discovering what the patient knows of his prognosis without directly asking him – which one may, for good reasons, be unwilling to do. The moral problem is that of whether one should give details of the patient's prognosis to other people, such as his social worker, without first ascertaining whether or not he knows these details himself (and informing him of them if it turns out that he does not), so that his permission to divulge them can be requested. At first sight the solution seems obvious: the patient should be approached and asked directly whether or not he knows that his condition is terminal, and then, in case he does not know, the full details of his condition should be laid before him. Only afterwards should the social worker be told the facts of the case. But what if the man's temperament is such that if he is now ignorant of the gravity of his condition, a sudden full disclosure of the facts, coming after a long period of medical and hospital treatment, would be profoundly disturbing for him? Is this a case in which it would be best to leave well alone and say nothing to the patient about his condition, while giving the full details to his social worker, despite the evident irregularity involved? Cases such as this are not uncommon in nursing: quite often, no-one seems to know exactly who has been told what, and an individual nurse may therefore wonder whether she should mention some detail of diagnosis or prognosis to a patient or one of his relations, because she cannot be certain that he already knows about it. But while some nurses can agonize over these decisions, others can treat them carelessly or fail to realise that they need to be made. The following report illustrates the difficulties which such negligence can cause:

> "One patient, Mrs. X, was admitted on several occasions, and at frequent intervals, for blood transfusions or treatment of infections arising from leukaemia. Her husband did not want his wife, who was only in her early 40s, to know the seriousness of her disease, and as a result the doctors had told her that she had a form of anaemia. During one of her stays in hospital after a severe infection had arisen, another patient was diagnosed as having carcinoma of the bronchus and was told of this. Being a very chatty person, she often wandered around the ward talking with the other patients, and one evening a nurse heard her saying to a group of patients that she had a similar problem to Mrs. X. Later this woman was reprimanded for her tactlessness by a Sister of the ward. But how could she have known that Mrs. X was unaware of her condition? And how did she find out about Mrs. X's condition in the first place? This seems to indicate an irresponsible action by the nursing staff, or medical staff, or both – i.e., talking about Mrs. X's leukaemia in the hearing of other patients. But it never became clear how and when this happened. Mrs. X was not told anything more about her condition and the whole incident seemed to be glossed over."

The view of the nurse recording this incident seems to be that the fault lay entirely with the nurse(s) and/or doctor(s) who had carelessly let slip remarks about Mrs. X's condition. But was it reasonable to expect that the truth would not eventually slip out, given that doctors and nurses do talk about their patients' conditions in the wards, where they can often be overheard? Should Mrs X's husband be criticized for demanding that hospital staff lie to Mrs. X? Certainly he should; but in this case it seems that the nurses should have refused from the start to take part in the subterfuge and urged that Mrs. X be told the truth. They should not have co-operated in such a subterfuge simply because Mr. X wanted them to do so.

(3) Handling confidential information concerning patients

In order to care for their patients, nurses need to have access to the facts about patients' conditions and prognoses. It is generally agreed that this sort of information should not be public knowledge, available to all and sundry, because it concerns intimate details of the patient's physical and mental condition, details which concern only him and the health professionals who are attempting to promote his recovery. An important parallel can be drawn between the patient's right to have this information regarded as confidential and his right to consent to or refuse treatment. For it is up to him whether or not a surgical operation or some other procedure is carried out on him, and the doctors and nurses who carry out the procedure do so only because he has requested this treatment, or because his consent to it can be reasonably presumed. Since, then, doctors and nurses treat or care for a patient only to the extent to which he authorizes them to do so, the information which they need if they are to care for him adequately is also something which comes their way only because he gives it to them. But "give" is a misleading word here. The patient does not give the information over to his doctors and nurses in the sense of actually transferring ownership of it from him to them. Rather, it still belongs entirely to him, the health professionals involved in his case being licensed only to make a limited use of it, namely, that use of it which is necessary for medical and nursing action on his behalf. Hence a doctor or nurse may not treat details of his or her patient's condition or prognosis as if it were entirely at his or her disposal: the health professional is the custodian of this information, not its owner.

If we ask "Why should details of a patient's condition and prospects be respected as confidential?", there seem to be two quite distinct arguments available. The first is just the argument set out above, that the information involved is the property of the patient and is only "lent", not strictly "given", to health professionals. This talk about "ownership" and "lending" is, of course, metaphorical, but it does express an important truth, namely that the information acquired by nurses and doctors is available to them only because the patient makes it available for strictly limited purposes. Many texts of bioethics have employed this terminology of "ownership", as, for example, T. J. O'Donnell in his *Morals in Medicine*. O'Donnell distinguishes various types of confidential information, or various kinds of "secret", as he calls it. One type is the natural secret, which holds in the absence of any formal agreement or contract, and another is the professional secret, in which (as in medicine and nursing) two parties enter into a contract binding one party, either explicitly or implicitly, to respect confidential information about the other party. O'Donnell then states:

> The secret, as a natural secret, is the property of the patient, and when the patient makes his secret known to the doctor he does not renounce his title to that property. Because of the implicit contract of the professional relationship, he merely assigns a limited use of that property to the professional person; namely, that use and only that use which the professional person has to make of the secret knowledge in order that he may accomplish the purpose for which the patient entered into the professional relationship with him.[1]

This argument appears to be reasonable. For, given that nurses and doctors can act only on their patient's behalf, he can legitimately be said to "own" the information which he gives to the health professionals. He can also, in a sense, be said to "own" the information yielded by the various tests and procedures which he undergoes, since the tests are carried out only because he consents to them. Admittedly, the medical and nursing records are legally the property of the hospital or other establishment at which the patient is treated; but this does not mean that the hospital owns the information contained in those records in such a way that the hospital authorities could divulge the information freely, without having to consider the patient's view of the matter. On the contrary, any attempt to divulge information about the patient will have to be justified on the grounds that the patient could be reasonably presumed to consent to it. So we find the UKCC making the point that

> The organisations which employ professional staff who make records (whether in the National Health Service or in other spheres of practice) are the legal owner of such records, but such ownership

---

1. T. J. O'Donnell, *Morals in Medicine*, p. 326.

does not give them any legal right of access to the information contained in those records. The patient also is involved in the ownership. The ownership of a record is therefore irrelevant to the patient's right of confidentiality and his/her expectation that personal health information will not be disclosed without consent.[1]

The second argument for regarding information about a patient's condition and prospects as confidential amounts to an appeal to the principle of respect for persons. For given that the patient *is* a person, it would be inappropriate to handle information about his condition in the way that one would handle (say) a report on the performance of a new model car. And the information contained in hospital records is not appropriate material for idle conversation but concerns matters of enormous personal importance to the patient. So a health professional must respect the patient as a person by using the information which he has supplied only for the good of the patient himself – and this will involve refraining from any disclosure of such information which is not ultimately related to this goal of promoting the patient's own well-being.

The crucial ethical questions concerning confidentiality seem to be as follows. Is it ever permissible to breach the requirement that one may not disclose confidential information? If so, when? And why should these exceptions to the general rule be permitted?

First, may one ever breach the requirement of confidentiality? The answer appears to be Yes: the requirement that confidential information be kept secret is not an absolute requirement which binds an agent come what may, as the prohibition against lying excludes all lies. The reason for this is that although lying is an act which of itself attacks the relationship which should hold between human thought and speech, the disclosure of a confidence does not *necessarily* undermine any basic good of human nature but may sometimes contribute to promoting people's genuine flourishing. The State, for instance, may require that certain information be made public in a court of law. Would it be permissible to supply the confidential information as evidence in a legal case, even against the patient's will? If we develop a little further the idea of confidential information as being the property of the patient, we see that it would be right to do this. For in general the right of an owner to do what he likes with his own property is subject to severe limitations, and sometimes

---

[1] UKCC, *Confidentiality: A UKCC Advisory Paper* (London 1987), p. 8.

individuals or the State will act rightly in using that property without first obtaining the owner's permission. (For example, in an emergency I run across someone's farm in order to reach a public telephone box from which I can summon an ambulance; the State issues a compulsory purchase order on some buildings so that they can be demolished and a new road constructed.) Individuals do have a right to use their own property as they wish, but that right is not absolute. For private property exists to serve not merely the good of the person who owns it, but the good of society in general: hence there can be occasions in which, if the public good as a whole requires it, one can rightly use the property of others in a way which would ordinarily be wrong; and the State may sometimes be justified in intervening, again on behalf of the public good, to regulate the use of someone's property in a way which he would disapprove. Likewise, then, an individual's right to have information concerning himself regarded as confidential may be overridden if the State requires that information to be made public in a legal action, and for a number of other reasons. As the UKCC's advisory paper on confidentiality points out:

'Confidentiality' is a rule with certain exceptions. . .

The needs of the community can, on occasions, take precedence over the individual's rights as for example in those situations where a court rules that the administration of justice demands that a professional confidence be broken or the law requires that patient confidence be breached.[1]

The general rule, then, is that the information which a patient supplies about himself is confidential information and must be kept confidential by the health professionals to whom it has been entrusted. But there are exceptions to this principle, just as there are to the principle that other people's property is not to be interfered with, and to the principle that promises are to be kept. What are these exceptions?

Clearly one such exception obtains when the patient himself gives permission for the information to be used in ways which would otherwise breach the requirement of confidentiality. Since the information is the property of the patient, he has the power to share it as widely or as narrowly as he wishes. Secondly, even when the patient has not expressly given permission for the information to be more widely shared, that

---

[1]. UKCC, *Confidentiality*, p. 10.

permission can sometimes be reasonably presumed. If, for instance, a hospital consultant has to consult another specialist about his patient's care and it would be impractical to obtain the patient's consent for this, he would act reasonably in presuming his consent. After all, the consultant's purpose in talking with the other specialist is to promote his patient's well-being, and this is the very same purpose as that for which the patient gave the information to him in the first place. So it is certainly reasonable to suppose that the patient would consent to the sharing of the confidential details if he were asked.

Some other proposed exceptions to the principle of confidentiality are, however, more controversial. Suppose that a nurse has to compile statistics from patients' records, in order to complete a nursing research project. May she go ahead and collect the statistics by examining patients' records, then forwarding them to the person in charge of the research project? Or does she need to obtain the consent of each individual patient before doing this? Here it seems that since the nurse is required only to collect the appropriate statistics and not to disclose the names of those whose records she has consulted, there is no real breach of confidentiality taking place. In any case, it will often be a reasonable supposition here that the patients themselves, if asked whether they would consent to their records being used for this purpose, would readily give permission. Nevertheless, the patients should surely be asked, if this is at all possible.

A much more difficult case is that in which the nurse, rather than obtaining the statistics herself, hands over the patient's records to a team of researchers so that they can work out the appropriate statistics. Such a move would amount to delivering the patient's records into the hands of people who play no part in caring for the patient. It is not difficult to see that the patient might understandably object to this use of his records, and so one certainly could not say here that his consent to the procedure could be reasonably presumed. Because of this, and because this is not one of those cases in which it is imperative that the individual's right to privacy be overridden in the interests of the public good, such a move must be condemned. The only proper course of action, in this sort of case, is to ask the patient whether he will allow his records to be used for the purposes of this research project. If he replies "No", that is the end of the matter: the records may not be used.

Some contemporary guidelines used in the handling of confidential material appear to transgress the ethical principles defended here. So great is the demand for suitable material for medical research that there is a constant temptation to "cut corners" by taking liberties with patients' rights to have confidences respected. So we find that a new draft code on confidentiality, issued by the Department of Health and Social Security, has received sharp criticism from the UKCC and the Royal College of Nursing on the grounds that it is "too ambiguously worded and too vague to protect the rights of patients".[1] The UKCC's director of professional conduct is quoted as objecting that "Information about health care would be too easy to release and [that] the code did not start from the premise that consent should always be sought". The report goes on:

> The UKCC is particularly worried about the code's guidance on the disclosure of health information without consent for medical research.

> The guidance, it says, "seems to start from the assumption that disclosure is acceptable as normal unless somebody stops you" – an approach which flies in the face of its own code of professional conduct.[2]

If we look at the handbook of professional ethics issued by the General Medical Council we see that there also, certain exceptions to the requirement of confidentiality are listed which it is difficult to justify. The GMC's handbook lists, in fact, eight kinds of exception to the requirement of confidentiality. These are:

(a) when the patient "or his legal advisor" gives written and valid consent;

(b) when other doctors or other health professionals are participating in the patient's care;

(c) when the doctor believes that a close relative or friend should know about the patient's health but it is medically undesirable to seek the patient's consent;

[1.] "UKCC upset at new confidentiality code", in *Nursing Times*, vol. 83, no. 32 (August 12–18, 1987), p. 6.
[2.] *Ibid.*

(d) exceptionally when the doctor believes that disclosure to a third party other than a relative would be in the "best interests of the patient" and when the patient has rejected "every reasonable effort to persuade";

(e) when there are statutory requirements to disclose information;

(f) when a judge or equivalent legal authority directs a doctor to disclose confidential medical information;

(g) (rarely) when the public interest overrides the duty of confidentiality "such as for example investigation by the police of a grave or very serious crime"; and

(h) for the purposes of medical research approved by a "recognised ethical committee".[1]

Some of these proposed exceptions are more obviously acceptable than others: (a), (e), (f) and (g), for instance, may clearly be accepted in the light of the basic principles argued for here. (b) seems acceptable also, given that the situation envisaged is team care for the patient, involving a number of doctors, possibly from a variety of specialities, who cannot treat him properly unless they share information. (c) and (d) are, however, more dubious, and could amount to an unjustifiable act of medical paternalism. As for (h), here we have an evidently immoral recommendation. The fact that a given programme of research has been approved by a "recognised ethical committee" cannot justify health professionals in enlisting patients as participants in that programme without the patients' express permission. To act in this way would be to fail to treat the patients with the respect to which, as persons, they are entitled.[2] Given that it would be wrong to subject a patient to participation in a programme of medical or nursing research without his knowledge and approval, it follows that a nurse should not co-operate in such programmes by handing over the patient's records to researchers or in any other way.

---

[1] General Medical Council, *Professional conduct and disciplines: fitness to practise* (London, 1985), pp. 19–21, quoted in R Gillon, *Philosophical Medical Ethics* (Chichester, 1986), pp.110–111.

[2] R. Gillon comments that requesting such permission from patients could be a simple matter: "This could be done routinely on admission or acceptance to a general practitioner's list and the files flagged accordingly." (*Philosophical Medical Ethics*, p. 111.)

(4) Truth-telling in obtaining consent for treatment

If a patient is to make an intelligent decision for or against treatment, he must be given the requisite information by the health professional involved, particularly the doctor. The doctor acts wrongly, then, if he hides some facts from the patient in order to make it more likely that he will agree to treatment. This is precisely what happened in the following incident at a hospital in the Republic of Ireland:

> A woman had been admitted to hospital for treatment of a cancer and had had some radium therapy which had not been entirely successful. Her doctor had therefore decided that chemotherapy should be tried, and had told the nurses who were caring for the patient that he would be approaching her to obtain her consent for the new course of treatment. After the doctor had been to speak with the woman, one of the nurses approached her and asked: "Well, did you agree to the chemotherapy?" At this the woman became extremely distressed and broke down. It appeared that the doctor had not mentioned the word "chemotherapy" in his discussion with her, but had simply talked in vague terms about alternative ways of tackling her problem and had got her to agree that she should "be open to other forms of treatment". He had said nothing definite about what specifically he had in mind or when he would want the new treatment to commence; but the nurse knew that he intended the chemotherapy to begin as soon as possible.

In this case, apparently, the doctor wanted to gain the patient's consent to chemotherapy without giving her any accurate information about what she would be letting herself in for, and, indeed, without even making it clear that he had come to see her precisely in order to secure her consent for a specific new form of treatment. The doctor had, then, failed in his duty to be completely frank with his patient, to lay before her the facts of the treatment she was being asked to undergo, the reasons for the treatment, its likely side-effects and its long-term consequences. The nurse is faced with the problem of deciding whether or not she should try to have the matter rectified. If she does resolve to take action she will have to decide on what steps to take: she may want to approach the doctor herself, or to put the matter in the hands of the ward sister, or, instead, simply to talk it over with her patient. If she takes the last of these three options, she will do so in the hope that the patient will decide either, on the one hand, to accept the idea of undergoing chemotherapy or, on the other, to seek a new meeting with the doctor in order to talk over the issue with him.

The administration of placebos

Two distinct issues are raised by the administration of placebos. First, is the practice itself morally legitimate? For the giving of placebos always involves some deception, since they are effective only to the extent that patients believe them to contain biochemically active ingredients, and one may question whether this deception of patients can be morally proper. Secondly, even if the general practice of giving placebos is unexceptionable, problems arise when patients ask nurses what it is that they are being given. One thing is certain: if the placebo is to have its desired effect, the nurse cannot respond to the patient's question by telling him the plain unvarnished truth, that is, by revealing that it is a placebo.

While these problems have caused headaches for some commentators on bioethical matters, they are not, perhaps, quite as intractable as they seem. The important point is that a placebo is prescribed for a patient because it is believed that it may benefit him; the fact that if it does benefit him it will be because of his own confidence in its supposed intrinsic powers is neither here nor there. Given that this sort of psychosomatic effect does take place, there seems to be no reason why the health professional should not take advantage of it in attempting to realize his overriding goal, that of assisting the patient's restoration to health. What, then, must a nurse say if her patient asks her about the nature of what is in fact a placebo? She may not, of course, lie to the patient by saying that the injection contains ingredients which it does not. But there is surely no objection to her telling the patient something less than the full truth ("It's something which will help you to overcome your persistent headaches"). As long as no lie is told to the patient, no wrong act is committed by the nurse. Of course, if the patient insists on knowing the exact ingredients of the "medicine" then he must be told the truth. In this case one will have to abandon all thought of using "the placebo effect" for the patient's good; but cases in which patients show such keen interest in the actual composition of their prescribed medicines will probably be rare.

The situation becomes more complex and dubious, however, when we consider placebos administered not in order to benefit a patient but as part of a controlled clinical trial of a new drug. It was argued in Chapter Eight that this way of treating patients is morally acceptable only if they have been informed of the possibility that they will be given a placebo and have consented to take part in the trial. For since the patient has contracted with health professionals only to receive medical treatment and nursing care designed to restore him to health, he has not given permission for any such non-therapeutic measures to be carried out on him. A second objection to this sort of procedure is that if a patient is made part of a control group and is denied, for experimental purposes, some treatment which would benefit him and which is being given to those outside the control group, we have a failure by health professionals to fulfil their side of the contract made with the patient: they would be doing less than they could reasonably be expected to do to bring about the patient's restoration to health. This sort of experimental programme could not be justified in terms of its beneficial consequences for other patients in the long term, for this would amount to using the patients being experimented upon as means to the welfare of others, and thus failing to give them that respect which they deserve as persons.

★   ★   ★

This Chapter in Summary

The heading "Problems of Honesty and Confidentiality" covers a wide range of ethical problems, but the principal such problem is that of whether it is ever right to lie to someone: the way in which one answers this question will strongly influence one's approach to all the issues discussed here. There appear to be good grounds for concluding that lying is in principle wrong and should not be engaged in whatever the circumstances – even though some widely-accepted arguments to this effect are unconvincing. If this is correct, it will follow that nurses may not lie to patients about their prognoses, and this conclusion will in no way be affected by the fact that such a course of action may have been ordered by the patient's physician. This general prohibition against lying, together with considerations of the patient's dignity as a person, has implications for the way in which nurses should approach problems concerning the handling of confidential information and the use of placebos.

CHAPTER TEN

PROBLEMS OF LIFE AND DEATH – (1)

Ethical difficulties in which someone's life is at stake are of the utmost gravity. There seem to be five key problem areas which come under the heading "life-and-death problems", each of them distinguished from the others by the state or condition of the person whose life is at stake. If the person is an unborn child, we have the problem of abortion. For a nurse, this problem is likely to take the form of whether she should co-operate, and if so under what circumstances and to what extent, in abortion procedures. Secondly, if the person whose life is at stake is a defective new-born infant, one will have to ask whether, and under what circum- stances, the obligation to provide life-sustaining treatment holds or ceases to hold. The final clinical decisions on matters of this sort are made by hospital paediatricians, but, once again, nurses may be faced with some very severe problems of co-operation. Thirdly, a decision may have to be made concerning a terminally-ill patient, or one who has suffered fatal injuries: are doctors and nurses obliged to do everything they can to keep him alive? Fourthly, we have the problem of the debilitated elderly patient – one who is not terminally ill but is inevitably declining and weakening as he approaches the end of his life – about whom this same question arises: When may one cease striving to keep alive? And finally, there is the case of a person who regards his life as worthless and wishes to die, and who wants his doctor or nurse to take action to end his life. This case presents the problem of euthanasia, and a nurse may worry about the extent to which (if at all) she should appear to condone, or act in accordance with, a patient's apparent desire to be killed.

Any one of the five kinds of life-or-death problem might be considered before the others, but I shall deal first with the issue of *euthanasia*, because this issue raises particularly clearly the ethical problems involved in taking the life of a human being. In this chapter, therefore, we consider euthanasia and also the issue of treating debilitated elderly patients. Since this latter issue can be handled adequately only on the basis of a distinc- tion, standard in natural-law ethics, between ordinary and extraordinary means of preserving life, the next chapter is devoted to outlining and applying this distinction. Another issue for which the distinction between ordinary and extraordinary means is important, the treatment of the terminally ill and fatally injured, will also be considered in Chapter Twelve. In Chapter Thirteen the two remaining types of life-and-death problem, those concerning abortion and treatment of the handicapped new-born, will be considered.

The problem of euthanasia

The word "euthanasia" signifies the deliberate killing of people with the intention that they be spared great pain, suffering, loneliness, or, in general, a supposedly meaningless or worthless life. Proponents of euthanasia would claim that if a person – an elderly disabled man or woman, for instance – is so tormented by mental or physical suffering, or, perhaps, by sheer boredom, that he or she evidently fails to find life worthwhile, then it is morally permissible, and should also be legally permissible, to kill him or her. Some people argue that just as we would condemn as cruel and unfeeling a man who was able but unwilling to put a suffering animal out of its misery, so we should condemn those who could relieve the sufferings and unhappiness of hopelessly ill or disabled people by killing them but who refuse to do so.[1] At present, most advocates of euthanasia are prepared to defend only voluntary euthanasia (in which the person whose life is being ended consents to being killed), and would not attempt to defend or promote involuntary euthanasia (in which the killing is performed without the subject's consent, or even against his expressed wishes). Opponents of euthanasia sometimes argue that the underlying logic of the pro-euthanasia position commits those who hold it to favouring involuntary euthanasia as well; but however this may be, many ethical theorists, and especially Christian moralists, have insisted that *all* types of euthanasia, voluntary as well as involuntary, are

---

[1] Professor Antony Flew, for instance, remarks: "Our first main positive argument [*sc.* for legalizing euthanasia] opposes the present state of the law, and of the public opinion which tolerates it, as cruel. Often and appositely this argument is supported by contrasting the tenderness which rightly insists that on occasion dogs and horses must be put out of their misery, with the stubborn refusal in any circumstances to permit one person to assist another in cutting short his suffering. The cry is raised, 'But people are not animals!' Indeed they are not. Yet this is precisely not a ground for treating people worse than brute animals. Animals are like people, in that they too can suffer. It is for this reason that both can have a claim on our pity and our mercy." (A. G. N. Flew, "The Principle of Euthanasia", in A. B. Downing and Barbara Smoker (eds.), *Voluntary Euthanasia: Experts Debate the Right to Die* (London, 1986), pp. 43–4.)

immoral. We need to ask whether this attitude is rationally justifiable – whether, that is, there are sound reasons for regarding all euthanasiast acts as immoral.

The word "euthanasia" means "a good death", and much of the pressure for legalization of voluntary euthanasia has come from people who have been struck by the fact that the deaths of so many people are painful, drawn-out and apparently meaningless. Thus Dr. Leonard Colebrook, a former chairman of the Euthanasia Society, had this to say about the sufferings of many dying people:

> In addition to pain many of the unhappy victims of cancer have to endure the mental misery associated with the presence of a foul fungating growth; of slow starvation owing to difficulty in swallowing; of painful and very frequent micturition; of obstruction of the bowels; of incontinence; and of the utter prostration that makes of each day and night a 'death in life' as the famous physician, the late Sir William Osler, described it.

> Diseases of the nervous system in their turn lead all too often to crippling paralysis or inability to walk; to severe headaches; to blindness; to the misery of incontinence and bedsores. Distressing mental disturbances are often added to these troubles.

> Bronchitis, too, with its interminable cough and progressive shortness of breath, can have its special terrors, which medical treatment in the late stages can do little to abate.

> All these, and many other grievous ills which may beset the road to death, are often borne with great courage and patience – even when the burden is many times heavier by reason of loneliness and/or poverty... Medical progress has done much to alleviate suffering during the past century, but, in honesty, it must be admitted that the process of dying is still very often an ugly business.[1]

The picture painted by Dr. Colebrook is by no means applicable to the bulk of old people, and it could be argued that he exaggerates the degree of pain, discomfort, depression and hopelessness which typically attends the process of dying in the elderly. However, we cannot dismiss his

---

[1] Quoted in A. B. Downing, "Euthanasia: the Human Context", in Downing and Smoker, *Voluntary Euthanasia*, pp. 22–3.

description as inapplicable or his proposal for dealing with the problem, namely, legalized voluntary euthanasia, as totally groundless. For it is true that for some people the process of dying is so filled with pain and discomfort, and so devoid of any interest or enjoyment or diversion, that we can easily understand such a person's saying to himself: "What have I got to live for? Why should I want to go on living in this sort of way, since life for me now is continuous torment? Nothing is to be gained, surely, by 'hanging on' day after day, only to suffer more of the same. The only sensible thing to do is to end it as quickly as possible."

The principal argument in favour of voluntary euthanasia is a simple appeal to the practical consequences of allowing euthanasia at the patient's request. If we allow people to have their own deaths brought about, so the argument goes, we will thereby eliminate a great deal of pain, discomfort, depression and mental anguish which, at present, many people experience during the final weeks or months or even years of their lives. A utilitarian thinker would therefore probably regard the issue as an open-and-shut case. On the one hand, he would say, we have all the suffering which is now experienced by the dying, due to the fact that legal euthanasia is not yet an option; on the other hand we have the removal of all this suffering by the simple expedient of making euthanasia available to these people. Since the advantages are all on one side, it is clear that the only morally acceptable option is to remove the legal curbs on voluntary euthanasia. We can see, then, why some advocates of legalized euthanasia consider their case to be so compelling that only those whose minds are (as they see it) under the sway of religious and ethical prejudices could reject it.

Some clarifications

Two aspects of this argument for free recourse to voluntary euthanasia need to be clarified before we move on to assess the argument.

(1) Advocates of voluntary euthanasia often support their case by concentrating on the problems of elderly people whose desire to live has been undermined by illness, pain and discomfort, and in this chapter I shall also be preoccupied mainly with this group of people and their problems. But people of all ages can be considered appropriate subjects for euthanasia. A man of 40, let us say, is suffering from cancer of the throat which prevents him from breathing and eating normally, so that he must rely on special respiratory and feeding apparatus. Moreover, he is

continuously sedated in order to suppress pain, and he appears to take no pleasure in anything that he experiences. Evidently someone in this condition would be as appropriate a candidate for euthanasia as an elderly person who has to endure severe pain and discomfort and general misery. In this section on euthanasia I am concentrating above all on problems of elderly people whose lives are apparently devoid of any meaning or purpose, simply because these problems are among the most likely to give rise to pro-euthanasia sentiment. My overriding aim is to decide whether or not voluntary euthanasia can ever be morally justified; if the answer is in the negative, it will then be possible to approach the remaining life-and-death problems secure in the knowledge that one answer which is favoured by some people has to be ruled out of consideration.

(2) An opponent of euthanasia may object to the practice on one or both of two grounds. First, he may argue on utilitarian grounds that it is the maintenance of the moral or legal prohibition of euthanasia, not the removal of that prohibition, which promises the most beneficial consequences for society at large. It has sometimes been argued, for instance, that any widespread acceptance of voluntary euthanasia would impose strong pressure upon old people to request euthanasia out of consideration for their relations, and would also undermine people's respect for and confidence in the medical and nursing professions. It is also claimed that those who come to approve of voluntary euthanasia will be unable to hold the line there but will inevitably be led to approve *in*voluntary euthanasia under certain conditions, as well as various other death-dealing practices.[1] This is evidently a "slippery-slope" type of argument, and although such arguments are often treated with some ridicule by those who are pushing for change, there are indications that this particular slippery slope is real – that is, that if euthanasia is legalized, even under restrictive conditions, its widespread availability could result in a blunting of people's moral sensibilities in the matter of deliberate killing, so that they are able to approve of, and even take part in, killings which they would previously have condemned. This *may* partially explain the action of the four Dutch nurses who were arrested in 1987 on a charge of killing a young comatose patient by injecting him with a lethal dose of insulin. It is arguable that the fact that voluntary euthanasia has, as a result of a number

---

[1] Arguments along these lines are to be found in Professor Yale Kamisar's article "Euthanasia Legislation: Some Non-Religious Objections", in Downing and Smoker (eds.), *Voluntary Euthanasia*, pp. 110–154.

of judicial rulings, become common medical practice in certain circumstances in Holland may have created a climate in which health professionals feel justified in engaging in acts of involuntary (and therefore illegal) euthanasia.[1] The nurses are said to have defended their action on the grounds that the patient "had no chance of recovery, that further medical treatment would not benefit the boy and could even be called maltreatment".[2] But there is a world of difference between discontinuing treatment which is futile and actively killing a person. Whether the widespread practice of euthanasia in Holland was a factor in bringing these nurses to decide to kill their patient is naturally uncertain; but the idea that there could be a "slippery slope" of this kind deserves to be taken seriously.[3]

However, one may object to euthanasia not on any utilitarian grounds but simply on the grounds that the practice itself, regardless of its consequences, is immoral. Such an objection would cut no ice with someone wedded to a utilitarian theory of morality, but, as we have seen, utilitarianism is to be rejected. The principal objection to utilitarianism is precisely that there are certain types of human action which *in themselves*, and not on account of their consequences, are immoral and therefore not to be done under any circumstances. Since, in general, there are such intrinsically evil acts, we have to ask whether euthanasia is one of them.

Euthanasia as intrinsically wrong

Is euthanasia an intrinsically immoral act? There are two different arguments which might be taken to show this. The first argument is that since euthanasia involves the direct killing of an innocent human being it amounts to a direct attack upon one of the basic goods of human nature, the good of life, in the person of the one who is killed. The fact that the person killed himself requests death in no way weakens this conclusion, nor does it do anything to justify the action of the one who kills. Since it is always wrong to act directly against any of the basic goods, all euthanasiast acts can be ruled out.

---

[1]   See the report of this case in the *Nursing Times*, vol. 83, no. 12, 25 March, 1987, p. 8 ("Dutch Nurses in Euthanasia Drama").

[2]   *ibid.*

[3]   A recent report records that "It is estimated that between 2,000 and 6,000 cases of euthanasia are performed in Holland each year". (P. Darbyshire, "Whose Life? Whose Decision?", *Nursing Times*, vol. 83, no. 45, 11 November, 1987, pp. 27–29, at p. 29.)

This argument may well be sound, but it is open to an objection arising from conclusions reached in Chapter Six above. It was concluded there that the existence of a long-standing Christian tradition allowing killing in certain circumstances – particularly capital punishment and some killings in war – means that we cannot say that the deliberate killing of a human being is always immoral. The advocate of euthanasia might ask, therefore: "Since you are prepared to admit the possibility that killing can sometimes be justified in these two cases, why not admit that it can be justified when death is sought by a patient on the grounds that he no longer wishes to live?" It may be replied that euthanasia involves the deliberate killing of an *innocent* human being and that this sets it apart as something which is always intrinsically evil. But it is doubtful whether the principle appealed to here – that the deliberate killing of innocent human beings is wrong – can be supported *solely* on the grounds that it involves directly attacking a basic human good. It was argued in Chapter Six that to show that the killing of innocent people is wrong we may have to consider explicitly the relationship between man and God, and in particular the distinction between God's absolute dominion over all creation, and, by contrast, man's strictly limited dominion. On this view, to seek to bring about death, either for oneself or for other people, is to attempt to take for oneself an absolute dominion over human life which belongs not to man but only to God. Man has no more than a strictly limited dominion over the lives of creatures, one which does not extend to innocent human beings. So a patient would act wrongly in trying to persuade his physician to give him a lethal injection, since his intention would be to have his own death brought about. Likewise, a doctor who deliberately gave a patient a lethal injection would be intending that the patient die and would thereby be acting wrongly – and it would make no moral difference whether the patient had consented to receiving the injection or not. Again, if a nurse were to assist a doctor in carrying out a procedure which she knew to be aimed at ending a patient's life, she would be sharing in the doctor's intention that the patient die; that is, she would be co-operating formally with him in his evil action, and her conduct would be every bit as immoral as his.

The conclusion defended here – that it is not up to man to take innocent human life and that in these matters he must act always in a way which respects God's absolute dominion over creation – is clearly in accord with the outlook expressed in the Scriptures. Some recent observations of a Christian geriatrician are worth quoting:

In the Old Testament, Elijah, in the midst of his depression, not to mention his physical and emotional exhaustion, asks the Lord for 'euthanasia' – 'It is enough – take away my life!' (1 Kings 19: 3). His request was not denied – it was simply ignored! He was fed, rested, ministered to, and then sent off to a further realm of fruitful service.

In the first chapter of II Samuel, an Amalekite makes the claim that he administered euthanasia to Saul in his mortally wounded state, Saul having already asked his armour-bearer to do the same for him. The response to this claim makes it quite clear that this was not an acceptable action, even in the heat of battle and in the case of severe, possibly mortal, wounds.

When we turn to the New Testament we find the Lord Jesus Christ bringing some to life from death, and bringing healing to many more, but we nowhere read of him bestowing the gift of death to a sufferer whose condition was intractable or irremediable. For him personally, death was an enemy to be finally defeated. Although it was to be the means to the glorious end, his resurrection, he did not embrace it without that horror and abhorrence which we glimpse in the Garden of Gethsemane.[1]

Someone who accepts that God exists and that His relationship with the created world is as the Christian religion describes it will therefore realize that euthanasia, since it is a deliberate killing of an innocent human being, is always wrong. So once we have determined that a given action or programme of treatment amounts to euthanasia – once we have realized that the treatment is being given precisely in order to bring about someone's death – the moral question at issue can be resolved. The action is immoral because it consists in human beings attempting to take on an authority over life and death which does not belong to them.

To say this is not, of course, to deny the severity of the physical and mental sufferings which may lead many people to regard a quick, painless killing as the only sensible and really effective way out. Certainly such suffering can often be intense and apparently unrelieved by any elements, however small, of rest and enjoyment. But it is one thing to recognize the undoubtedly pitiable condition of many people in this state, and quite

---

1. G. Chalmers, "Life Issues: (3) Euthanasia", in I. L. Brown and N. M. de S. Cameron (eds.), *Medicine in Crisis: A Christian Response* (Edinburgh, 1988), pp. 102–119, at p. 116.

another to recommend that their problems be solved by killing them. Such a recommendation would amount to a proposal to do evil that good might come.

Here we have the first argument for the conclusion that euthanasia is always morally wrong. A disadvantage of this argument is that since it is explicitly based on considerations about the relationship of man to God and the contrast between God's absolute dominion over things and man's merely relative dominion, it can be persuasive only for those who believe in God. It can offer no reason to those with no settled religious convictions to reject euthanasia as always wrong. Can we state an argument which has a wider appeal than this one?

This brings us to the second argument for rejecting euthanasia as intrinsically wrong. The case *for* euthanasia is based on the claim that a person who is seriously injured or debilitated or suffering from great pain may have a life whose quality is so diminished that it is not worth living. That person would then have a "worthless" or "valueless" life. Precisely because his life would have no value, the moral norms prohibiting killing would be inapplicable in his case. Proponents of euthanasia usually claim that for euthanasia to be morally justified, it must be requested by the person whose life is thought valueless. It would be wrong, in other words, for doctors to kill someone without his consent on the grounds that his life is worthless. If he wants to continue living despite his intense suffering, that is up to him, and health professionals must respect his decision. On the other hand, a patient's request for euthanasia is not by itself sufficient to justify doctors and nurses in killing. There must also be a professional judgment to the effect that his life really is worthless and hence that his request for euthanasia is reasonable. This professional judgment would presumably be made by doctors, even though such an expansion of their role would be profoundly disturbing to many of them.[1]

The crucial question here is: Can this judgment, that a person's life is worthless, reasonably be made? If so, how, on what grounds? Advocates

---

[1] As G. Chalmers remarks: "The doctor, by virtue of his clinical relationship with his patient, is in a position of clear responsibility for the life and health of that patient, and it would be quite inimical to that responsibility for him to be 'licensed to kill'. Such a concept could only undermine and eventually destroy the basic confidence on which the doctor-patient relationship is built. . . 'Hanging judges' have been recognised in the past and are remembered with infamy: few practitioners would wish to be defined as 'killing doctors'." (*Medicine in Crisis: A Christian Response*, p. 10.)

of euthanasia often claim that the presence of intense and lasting pain, severe depression together with a general feeling of hopelessness, or greatly diminished mental powers – or, of course, a combination of all these – may be sufficient to make this judgment reasonable. Clearly what lies behind such a claim is a certain conception of human nature, of what sort of a being man is and what sorts of activities are "natural" and worthwhile to him. It is assumed that what gives meaning and value to human existence is the ability to engage in certain conscious activities, involving the use of intelligence and reason – such activities as talking to other people, thinking about various matters, enjoying various experiences provided by one's senses, and so on – unimpeded by such factors as intense pain or infirmity or depression. This sort of picture of what human life is all about is often taken for granted by supporters of euthanasia, and admittedly it contains elements of truth. Given that (as argued in Chapter Five above) such goods as knowledge, play and aesthetic appreciation really are basic goods of human nature, someone whose participation in these goods is largely destroyed by intense pain or severe injury is certainly suffering impairment to his flourishing or fulfilment. However, to say this is not to say that human flourishing is completely *destroyed* when these sufferings are present, or that their presence renders one's life worthless or pointless. There are other goods than the ones mentioned, as, for example, the good of practical reasonableness; and even a person whose life is racked by pain and other sufferings may be able to participate in this good in a valuable way, simply by reflecting seriously on the way in which he should try to cope with his sufferings and put his affairs in order, and, in general, how he should order his life, particularly in relation to his loved ones, in the time that is left to him. One way of participating in the good of practical reasonableness is to come to realize the importance of *integrity* for man's moral life, the fact that in acting one makes oneself to be a person of a certain sort of moral character, and that to commit a morally evil act is to corrupt oneself. In realizing that this is so – that integrity is important for man, that it is itself a part of genuine human flourishing – we realize also that the sort of picture of the worthwhileness of human life on which advocates of euthanasia base their argument is seriously inadequate. To live in a worthwhile fashion consists not just in enjoying pleasurable experiences and being free from from pain and other suffering. A concern to do what is morally good and avoid evil, and in particular an awareness that one must never do evil that good may come, is also an essential part of human flourishing, and one which cannot be accommodated by the utilitarian criteria on which supporters of euthanasia usually base their calculations of the overall value of someone's life. Just as Socrates's decision not to assist in the judicial murder of Leon of Salamis is one which makes no sense on utilitarian presuppositions, so the conception of human well-being favoured by advocates of euthanasia has no obvious place for the moral integrity which grounded Socrates's decision. Admittedly, a person's mental powers may be so ravaged by great suffering that coherent thought about moral right and wrong, or awareness of the importance of integrity, may be impossible for him. The point is, however, that because integrity *is* of great importance for human flourishing (whether a given person is capable of realizing this or not) the picture of human flourishing which underlies euthanasiast arguments is false to the reality of human nature: by confining its attention to enjoyable and painful experiences it misses out on a whole dimension of human life. This dimension of human existence which advocates of euthanasia fail to recognize has been called a "dimension of spirit",[1] and the fact that man alone, among embodied creatures, possesses this "side" to his character is arguably what justifies us in putting animals, but not our fellow human beings, out of their misery.

For Christian believers the "dimension of spirit" which characterizes human beings will be manifested, above all, by the fact that we are created by God and destined for a life of communion with Him which begins while we are alive on earth but which continues and reaches its fulfilment after death. If this orientation to eternal life with God is indeed an aspect of what we ourselves are, it will persist in us no matter what sufferings we have to endure, and it will therefore be wrong to say that a person's life is not worthwhile, not of value. On the contrary, just because this "dimension of spirit" is an integral part of what man is, his life is *always* valuable. This means, not that one is always obliged to keep someone alive at all costs, but simply that if one decides not to do so, this decision must be taken not on the grounds that his life is lacking in value, but (say) on the grounds that continued treatment would be excessively burdensome to him. However, even if we put to one side specifically Christian ideas concerning man's orientation to a life of intimate friendship with God,

---

[1]   A. J. L. Gormally, "A nonutilitarian case against voluntary euthanasia", in Downing and Smoker (eds.), *Voluntary Euthanasia*, pp. 72–95.

there are other aspects of human nature which indicate that the sort of calculation on which the pro-euthanasia case is founded fails because it is based on a false estimation of what makes a human life worthwhile. One such aspect of human nature has already been mentioned: the moral integrity which is a key feature of our moral lives.

The argument is, then, that the advocate of euthanasia proceeds on the basis of an impoverished conception of human nature, he wrongly regards some human lives as lacking in value; hence he fails to make out a case that euthanasia may sometimes be justified. How effective is this argument? It certainly does show that the euthanasiast's conception of human nature is impoverished and that his criteria for deciding what is a worthwhile life are therefore unfounded. The advocate of euthanasia could, however, advance the following reply to the argument. "I concede your point that there's a 'dimension of spirit' in man which I haven't accommodated in my argument up to now. This 'dimension of spirit' is certainly a part of human nature which remains in people even when they are suffering great pain or mental and physical exhaustion, etc. However, suppose that someone's sufferings are so great, or that his condition has deteriorated to such an extent, that none of the activities which manifest this 'dimension of spirit' – conscientious moral judgment, for example – can possibly be exercised, either now or in the future. May we not then say that although this spiritual dimension remains in him in a potential, unactualized state, the fact that it can never again be expressed in action means that we may treat it in practice as if it did not exist? Surely a 'dimension of spirit' which exists in a latent state only and can never possibly be actualized is not really all that different from one which does not exist at all?"

This reply is a possible way out for the advocate of euthanasia. Clearly the debate would not stop at this point, because the opponent of euthanasia may have a reply to it; but I suspect that the argument on this issue would swing back and forth between supporters and opponents of euthanasia, with no conclusive result. To put the matter beyond doubt, I believe, we need to understand the "dimension of spirit" in human nature in a full sense, as referring to the orientation of man to a destiny extending beyond this earthly life and centring on an intimate friendship with God Himself. If this is really what human life is all about, then it is clearly the case that *any* human life, no matter how deprived or racked by suffering and misery, is intrinsically valuable, and may therefore not be terminated on the grounds that it is not worthwhile. Does this mean that this second line of objection to euthanasia, is, like the first argument, limited in its appeal to those who already believe in God? No, because the fact that there is a spiritual dimension in man's life of which euthanasiast calculation can take no account should lead supporters of euthanasia to question the value of their whole approach to the problem. They should ask themselves whether this spiritual dimension extends beyond the limited area which they have been forced to admit by a consideration of the importance of integrity in man's moral life. However, it does seem to me that while criticism of euthanasiast criteria for the value of a life may do much to weaken the confidence of supporters of euthanasia in their principal argument, a completely effective rebuttal of the euthanasiast argument comes only when we bring God into the picture and defend the idea that communion with God is one of the basic human goods. This does not mean that the opponent of euthanasia has nothing of value to say to the atheist or agnostic supporter of euthanasia; but it may be that the argument can be resolved *conclusively* only if it is based on God as provident creator of the universe and on man as orientated to a life of intimate friendship with God.

In practice, too, religious belief can be crucially important, because a person who regards himself as utterly dependent on God's providence and needing to direct himself always towards the goal of loving union with God may thereby be enabled to find meaning even in great suffering which would appear totally meaningless on a wholly this-worldly perspective. While one is naturally sceptical about generalized claims that suffering ennobles the sufferer, or that it is "good for the soul", it is certainly arguable that intense suffering *accepted in the right spirit* does confer great benefits upon the character of the sufferer. For a Christian, "the right spirit" will be a spirit of self-renunciation, of uniting oneself with Christ in His sufferings and offering up one's own sufferings and infirmities to be used by Him in the building-up of His Kingdom. So although the opponent of euthanasia has to combat the arguments proposed in favour of it and to defend his claim that any deliberate taking of a suffering person's life is immoral, he does not have to leave the matter at that. He can also dispute the claim that euthanasia manifestly secures the best consequences for all concerned; for he can point out that a person who approaches his sufferings in a spirit of union with the sufferings of Christ will see those sufferings not as utterly pointless and meaningless, but as capable of contributing – in ways which we cannot, of course, be expected to appreciate fully in this life – to the spiritual growth of the patient himself and of others with whom he is in contact. The Vatican's *Declaration on Euthanasia*, issued in 1980, expresses this idea clearly, and with a wise recognition of the limitations as well as the heroic capabilities of human beings:

> According to Christian teaching,... suffering, especially suffering during the last moments of life, has a special place in God's saving plan; it is in fact a sharing in Christ's passion and a union with the redeeming sacrifice which he offered in obedience to the Father's will. Therefore one must not be surprised if some Christians prefer to moderate their use of painkillers, in order to accept voluntarily at least a part of their sufferings and thus associate themselves in a conscious way with the sufferings of Christ crucified (cf. Matthew 27: 34). Nevertheless it would be imprudent to impose an heroic way of acting as a general rule. On the contrary, human and Christian prudence suggests for the majority of sick people the use of medicines capable of alleviating or suppressing pain, even though these may cause as a secondary effect semi-consciousness and reduced lucidity. As for those who are not in a state to express themselves, one can reasonably presume that they wish to take these painkillers, and have them administered according to the doctor's advice.

When is an act one of euthanasia?

Euthanasia is the deliberate killing of people who are judged (either by themselves or by others) not to have worthwhile lives. So, in deciding whether or not a given act is one of euthanasia, we have to judge whether it is a deliberate killing; and since this involves making judgments about people's intentions – about what they are aiming at or trying for in doing what they do – it will sometimes be difficult to decide whether we are dealing with a case of euthanasia or not. We must, nevertheless, do our best to answer such questions as "Is what Dr. X/Nurse Y proposes to do clearly aimed at ending the patient's life, or could it reasonably be taken to have some other point?"[1]

[1.] Sacred Congregation for the Doctrine of the Faith, *Declaration on Euthanasia* (Vatican City, 1980), p. 8.

The following situation, reported by a nurse working at a London hospital, illustrates the difficulty of deciding whether or not a proposed course of action would amount to euthanasia.

"A 77-year-old man had had arterial surgery and after the operation had simply given up the will to live. He refused to eat and had only little to drink. He told us that he had had a good life and had "had just enough" now after this big operation. He had also previously had a cerebro-vascular accident which had left him totally paralysed down one side. One night, after a whole day in which he had been becoming drowsier, he suddenly stopped breathing. There was a staff nurse and myself, and neither of us tried to resuscitate him as he had died so peacefully. The doctors were angry that we had not tried, after all their (and our) hard work to keep him alive; but the man had simply given up the will to live."

Was the man's attitude a euthanasiast one? It might be suggested that it was, on the grounds that if he had really given up the will to live, he had evidently decided that his life was no longer worth living and that it should be ended as soon as possible. But it is clear on reflexion that to impute this line of thought to him would be to read too much into his remarks. The most natural explanation of his words "I've just had enough" is that his energies were thoroughly depleted after all that he had been through, and that he was overcome by exhaustion and a feeling of hopelessness, as well as an aversion to continued medical treatment. There is no reason to think that he had judged his life to be not worth living or that he was seeking to have it ended.

Sometimes, however, a patient's motives in making certain requests of a doctor or nurse, or a health professional's motives in responding to changes in his or her patient's condition, would evidently be euthanasiast. Suppose that Mrs. Brown is suffering from an incurable disease which at present is not far advanced but will eventually make her unable to control her bodily movements and lead to loss of mental capacity, together with considerable pain and discomfort. Mrs. Brown regards life in such a condition as not worth living, and so she tries to persuade her doctor to bring it about that she will die before her condition deteriorates too far. Does Mrs. Brown's request amount to a request for euthanasia? Clearly it does, because the crux of the matter is that *she intends that her death be brought about*; and this intention is by definition a euthanasiast one. If she should persuade a doctor to facilitate her early death, the doctor would share that intention; and so would a nurse who knowingly and deliberately assisted the doctor in his killing of Mrs. Brown.

A question of terminology

Many writers distinguish between what they call active euthanasia and passive euthanasia. The former is the direct and deliberate killing of a patient by intervening in some way (e.g., by giving him a lethal injection), while the latter amounts to the withholding of treatment which would have prolonged a patient's life. It is sometimes said that while active euthanasia is always wrong, passive euthanasia can often be morally justified. The suggestion conveyed by the use of this distinction is that in both cases the same kind of act is performed, namely euthanasia, but that the way in which it is performed differs from one situation to the other. This suggestion should be resisted, because many acts of withholding treatment, since they do not proceed from an intention that a patient die (but rather, e.g., from an intention to avoid treatment which is futile or burdensome), do not amount to euthanasia at all. Some acts of withholding treatment *are* motivated by a death-dealing intention and hence are euthanasiast acts, but the fact that the term "passive euthanasia" covers acts of both these kinds, despite the important differences between them, means that it is an inevitably confusing piece of terminology which should not be used by someone who wants to think clearly about these matters.

The debilitated elderly patient

The question "When does an act of 'letting die' amount to euthanasia and when does it not?" is at stake in the problem of treatment of debilitated elderly patients. By "the debilitated elderly" I mean people who, while not in any immediate danger of death, are clearly declining towards death, and for whom any sufficiently severe physical or mental upset could trigger off a series of changes ending in death. They are not suffering simply from old age, but also from one or more supervening conditions which have served to weaken them seriously. A common ethical difficulty arises from the fact that debilitated elderly patients are prone to contract certain viral or bacterial infections, particularly pneumonia. In the not-too-distant past, before antibiotics had come into widespread use, these infections would often prove fatal, thus sparing these old people a long, drawn-out and painful death at a later stage. Now, however, antibiotics can be used to cure the infection and thus save the patient. A probable consequence of such treatment is that the patient, after being cured, will be even more debilitated, even more prone than before to contract potentially fatal infections or to succumb to other severe shocks to the system. Given that this is so, would a doctor sometimes be justified in deciding not to prescribe antibiotics for a patient who had contracted pneumonia, thus permitting him to die? Decisions along these lines are certainly common in hospitals and nursing homes. If a doctor may legitimately refrain from administering antibiotics in some cases, it will follow that a nurse may co-operate with his decision. On the other hand, if a doctor would act wrongly in withholding treatment for the pneumonia, then, it would seem, nurses would be justified in refusing to co-operate with his decision and in protesting against it. May a doctor legitimately make such a decision or not? And if so, just *how* debilitated does his patient have to be?

Having posed this question, there we must leave it for the time being. For in dealing with this problem we need to appeal to the distinction mentioned briefly at the outset of this chapter, between ordinary and extraordinary means of preserving life. After this distinction has been outlined, in the next chapter, we shall be in a better position to deal with problems concerning treatment of the debilitated elderly. In Chapter Twelve some further problems of life and death are considered, some of which (namely, those concerning treatment of handicapped new-born babies) also need to be viewed in the light of the distinction between ordinary and extraordinary means if they are to be satisfactorily treated.

★   ★   ★

This Chapter in Summary

We begin our treatment of life-and-death issues in this chapter with a consideration of euthanasia and treatment of the debilitated elderly. The second of these issues, however, can be handled satisfactorily only on the basis of the distinction between ordinary and extraordinary means of preserving life, which is outlined in the next chapter; so our attention here is centred mostly on euthanasia. Discussion of euthanasia is often confused by the use of a supposed distinction between "active" and "passive" euthanasia. But this distinction is itself groundless and misleading: euthanasia involves the deliberate bringing-about of someone's death, and it is unimportant whether this is achieved by direct killing or by omission of life-preserving treatment. Since euthanasia is a type of killing of an innocent person, it is wrong in principle. The same conclusion, that euthanasia is intrinsically wrong, can be reached if we reflect on the inadequacy of the conception of human nature which underlies euthanasiast attitudes, and which finds expression in the belief that certain human lives are not worth living. The most difficult ethical problems which arise concerning euthanasia typically involve deciding whether a certain sort of act which appears, at first sight, to be a euthanasiast act really is such.

CHAPTER ELEVEN

PROBLEMS OF LIFE AND DEATH – (2)

The distinction between ordinary and extraordinary means of preserving life has been used widely by moral philosophers and theologians in their treatment of crucial life-and-death problems. They have claimed that by using this distinction we can resolve many ethical difficulties which raise the question "When are we obliged to try to prolong someone's life, and when may we allow a person to die?" This distinction between ordinary and extraordinary means is, however, itself based on another important distinction, that between acts and omissions. This latter distinction will therefore be examined first.

Acts and omissions

In Chapter Seven it was argued that although one may not deliberately take the life of any innocent human being, nevertheless one may act in ways which result in someone's death if the conditions laid down in the principle of double effect apply. One of these conditions is that the person's death is not what one directly brings about but is rather a side-effect or after-effect of one's action. And, it was also argued, whether or not I directly bring about some result in action depends very largely upon what my intention *in* acting is: if I am not setting myself to bring it about that someone dies then I cannot be said to *kill* him, at least in the strict sense of these words, even though I may still act wrongly.

The fact that we must never intentionally take innocent human life does not mean that we must always do everything we possibly can to keep ourselves and other people alive. For although life is a basic human good it is not the only one; and by striving always and constantly to keep people alive we should inevitably be neglecting the pursuit of other basic goods. If, as Christians maintain, there is an afterlife, consisting in a condition of intimate friendship with God, to which man's life on earth is essentially orientated, an absolute concentration on preserving one's bodily life at all costs would even be detrimental to one's orientation to the ultimate end of human life, friendship with God. One could, in other words, be too solicitous or zealous in preserving one's life or the lives of other people. Here, as elsewhere, one needs moderation: one needs to know when to strive single-mindedly to keep alive, and when to "let go", so to speak. We are, then, in general obliged to promote and safeguard human life. But this obligation has limits, and there may be occasions on which we would be justified in not acting to defend or preserve life.

Can we conclude that while all acts of deliberate killing are wrong, by contrast all deliberate omissions which result in someone's death are morally blameless? Surely not; this would be to take an over-simple view of the act/omission distinction, because some omissions resulting in a person's death would be just as obviously cases of murder as a killing by active intervention. Suppose that a man drinks lemonade which I know to be poisoned, and that I stand by and let him drink it, even though I could easily stop him. (We assume here that there is no compelling reason for me to stay silent: I am not gagged or paralyzed, nobody is threatening me with death if I try to shout a warning, etc.) By acting in this way I should be morally responsible for the death of the poisoned man, because my inaction would be inexplicable unless I had wanted him dead and had intended that through my keeping silent he should die.

Therefore some omissions which result in a person's death will be cases of murder. But equally, some will not. Take the following case. A man whom I know to be innocent of any crime is awaiting execution under an unjust and malevolent regime. I could have him smuggled out of prison, but since I know that this could lead to my own execution I do not do so. As a result the prisoner is eventually put to death. Am I at fault in not sacrificing my life for this unjustly condemned man? Surely not. I deliberately omit to save his life, but this is because of a perfectly reasonable fear of losing my own life; I certainly in no way *intend* that he should die. Of course, I would not act wrongly by exposing myself to execution in order to set him free: this would be a praiseworthy act of supererogation, something "above and beyond the call of duty"; but the point is that the act *would* be one of supererogation, not of strict moral obligation.

Concerning the morality of omitting to save life as against directly taking life, we must, then, give the following verdict. First, *all* deliberate takings of innocent human life amount to murder; secondly, *some* cases of deliberately omitting to preserve innocent human life amount to murder, while some others do not.

The crucial question is, then: What distinguishes those omissions of life-saving or life-preserving action which amount to deliberate killing from those which do not? If we can find what this decisive criterion is, then, on the medical front, we shall be better able to decide which types of non-treatment decisions (that is, decisions either not to treat someone or to withdraw treatment once it has been started) may be justified.

The answer surely lies in the concept of intention, which we have already seen to be crucial for determining the moral status of human acts. For our acts and omissions are the kinds of acts and omissions which they are precisely because of the intentions involved in them. A human action is not a mere physical movement; it has a mental side as well as a physical side to it, and its mental side consists in one's knowledge of what one is doing and one's intention to do it. Likewise an omission, if it is a deliberate omission rather than an unthinking oversight, must have a mental as well as a physical aspect. My omitting to do something is not merely a matter of my not doing it; rather, to omit to do something which one is capable of doing, one must *intend* not to do it; so intention is an essential ingredient in omissions no less than in acts.

An act which results in someone's death will be an act of murder if I intend that that person die as a result of my act. However, a death-dealing intention can be present just as much in omissions as in acts; and an omission which expresses an intention that someone die will be just as evil as a positive act to kill. But here there is a crucial difference between acts and omissions. Every active killing will necessarily involve an intention that someone die. But some omissions will be motivated by quite different aims or intentions, even though they have the inevitable consequence that someone dies; in these situations, death will not be the result aimed at, and if it occurs it will be an unintended consequence or side-effect of one's omission. Provided that one's reasons for omitting to act are sound and sufficiently weighty, one will be justified in not acting. One will therefore foresee and tolerate the death of someone without causing it; or, to express things differently, one will not be killing but simply "letting die". It is, then, only by adverting to the element of intention that one can properly understand why the distinction between killing and letting die is crucially important from a moral point of view.[1]

---

[1]   For more detailed discussions of the significance of the distinction between killing and letting die, cf. J. M. Boyle, "On Killing and Letting Die", *The New Scholasticism*, vol. 51, 1977, pp. 433–53, and two publications of the Linacre Centre: *Prolongation of Life Paper 2: Is there a morally significant difference between killing and letting die?* (London, 1978) and *Euthanasia and Clinical Practice: The Report of a Working Party* (London, 1982), Chapter Three, pp. 24–36.

Ordinary and extraordinary means

Applying the principles stated above, we can say that if life-preserving treatment were to involve (e.g.) great pain or severe mutilation, a patient could be justified in rejecting that treatment, even though death would be a probable, or even inevitable, consequence of his decision. For his motive or intention would not be to bring about his death, but simply to avoid the great pain, suffering, inconvenience or mutilation involved in the treatment. In situations such as these, the means required for the preservation of life would be regarded as *extraordinary* means.

There are, in fact, two elements in the technical notion of extraordinariness as moralists have employed it. The first is that of *great burden or hardship*, and the second is that of *lack of genuine benefit*. If a particular type of proposed treatment displays either of these features – if it either involves unreasonably great hardship, either for the patient or for others, or if it fails to confer any genuine benefit on the patient – then it is regarded as extraordinary and therefore as not morally obligatory. By contrast, if a proposed treatment is both beneficial to the patient and free of any intolerably harmful side-effects or consequences it is an ordinary treatment and therefore morally obligatory.[1]

Consider the question of whether one should artificially ventilate a grossly defective newborn baby who has no prospects of living for more than a short time, whatever is done to him. Such treatment would plainly count as extraordinary since it is both productive of hardship (i.e., the discomfort of the ventilation itself) and lacking in any real benefit for the patient. (There may, however, be a sound reason for continuing artificial ventilation for some time – for example, so that the baby's parents will be able to visit and hold him and thus come to have that very limited knowledge of their child which is all that is possible in the circumstances.)

Another example would be the artificial ventilation of an irreversibly comatose patient. Here also it seems evident that no real benefit is conferred upon the patient, and although the operation of the ventilator

---

[1]   Cf. the summary definition given by G. Kelly, S.J., in his *Medico-Moral Problems*, pp. 134–5: A medicine, treatment, etc., is to be considered an ordinary means if it can be obtained and used with *relative convenience* and if it offers *reasonable hope of benefit*. When either of these conditions is lacking, the means is extraordinary. . . [In other words,] *extraordinary* means of preserving life are all medicines, treatments and operations which cannot be obtained or used without excessive expense, pain or other inconvenience for the patient or for others, or which, if used, would not offer a reasonable hope of benefit to the patient.

does not cause him any hardship, since he is unconscious, it may cause considerable hardship to others and be a severe strain on the financial and other resources of society at large.

Next, consider the amputation of the gangrenous leg of a man who is otherwise in good health. Provided that facilities are available for such a treatment (i.e., that the man is not living in a country where resources for surgery are primitive), amputation in these circumstances is unquestionably an ordinary means; for, given the quality of modern anaesthetic and surgical techniques, it does not cause great hardship to the patient, and the benefit to be derived from the operation – a lengthening of the patient's life, perhaps for many years – is substantial. However, suppose that the man with the gangrenous leg also has an overwhelming and uncontrollable fear of surgery (or, perhaps, of losing a limb): try as he might, he cannot tolerate the thought of submitting himself to the surgeon's knife, even though he knows that his days are numbered unless he does so. Natural-law moralists would regard this extreme fear of surgery as sufficient to constitute the operation an extraordinary means; they would therefore say that someone possessing this extreme and uncontrollable fear would not be obliged to undergo the treatment, even though the latter would be the only alternative to a rapid death. For the extreme mental upset occasioned by all thoughts of the coming operation would constitute a grave hardship for the patient. In a similar vein, theologians of the seventeenth and later centuries declared that someone who was so strongly attached to his own home or district as to dread being parted from it would not be obliged to move to another region with a healthier climate, even if, by staying at home, he were to suffer a much earlier death. So a certain treatment which, other things being equal, would be an ordinary means of preserving life, may be an extraordinary means in the case of some patients who have particular weaknesses and susceptibilities.

Some additional clarifications

The distinction between ordinary and extraordinary means is easily misunderstood, and some attacks which are commonly made upon it, by health professionals and also by writers on medical ethics, are evidently the result of misunderstanding. The following clarificatory points are therefore worth making.

(1) There is an important difference between the meanings of the words "ordinary" and "extraordinary" as used, on the one hand, by moralists in the natural-law tradition, and, on the other hand, by many health professionals, particularly physicians. The latter tend to take the literal meaning of "ordinary" as "commonplace" and of "extraordinary" as "unusual". If this way of understanding these terms is combined with a belief that ordinary means are morally obligatory whereas extraordinary means are not, the result is confused thinking in clinical decision-making. A treatment which is quite "ordinary" in the sense that it is performed very regularly and presents no great difficulties to medical and nursing staff (e.g., intravenous feeding) will nevertheless be extraordinary, in the strict ethical sense, for a patient who cannot derive any benefit from it; and likewise, some very rare and unusual treatments will have to be judged ordinary in the ethical sense for a particular patient because they benefit him significantly and can be provided without being a serious burden on him or anyone else.

This misunderstanding on the part of many doctors of what the distinction between ordinary and extraordinary means is all about is to some extent understandable, because the words "ordinary" and "extraordinary", in normal English usage, just do bear the respective meanings of "commonplace" and "exceptional/out of the ordinary". For this reason many defenders of the traditional principle have urged that while the distinction itself must be retained, the words "ordinary" and "extraordinary" should be scrapped in favour of alternatives which indicate more unambiguously what the distinction is about. Various alternative expressions have been proposed for this purpose. The President's Commission in the U.S.A. recommended the terms "proportionate care" and "disproportionate care",[1] while it has also been urged that "overtreatment" or "unjustified treatment" be substituted for "extraordinary means".[2] However, none of these proposed alternatives has caught on, and the phrases "ordinary means" and "extraordinary means" appear to be here to stay. In these circumstances, we seem forced to accept the continuing widespread use of these terms, despite the fact that they are liable to

---

[1] President's Commission, *Deciding to Forego Life-sustaining Treatment* (Washington, 1983), p. 82.

[2] N. Tonti-Filippini, "Overtreatment: An Ethical Viewpoint", in J. N. Santamaria and N. Tonti-Filippini (eds.), *Proceedings of the 1984 Conference on Bioethics* (Melbourne, St. Vincent's Bioethics Centre, n.d.), pp. 31–44.

mislead. The Vatican's *Declaration on Euthanasia* wisely insists on the substance of the principle rather than on the terms in which it is expressed.[1]

(2) The distinction between ordinary and extraordinary means was first developed, by scholastic theologians of the seventeenth century, to answer questions about the limits to the *competent* patient's obligation to take steps to preserve his own life. But the scope of the distinction can be extended to apply to the incompetent patient as well. The important thing here is that in deciding not to press for extraordinary means the proxy decision-makers must consider what it would be reasonable for the patient to choose, given his condition and the way in which treatment would be likely to affect him, mentally as well as physically. In addition, those who make the decision must seek to ensure that the patient is treated justly by health professionals, that he is not denied any treatment or assistance which he has a right to receive, or unfairly discriminated against in any way.

(3) The notions of ordinary means and extraordinary means are patient-dependent: what one person finds intolerable hardship another may not; and due to advances in medical techniques what will be intolerable hardship for almost everybody at one period of time (e.g., certain operations such as amputations) will not be so (and therefore will have become ordinary means) at other times.

(4) A closely-related point. There is no way of determining with quasi-mathematical precision whether a certain degree of hardship is intolerable or not. So in expounding the criterion of extraordinary means one is forced to employ vague-sounding phrases such as "*grave* hardship", "*intolerable* suffering", "*extremely serious* burden", and so on. Since there is no way of quantitatively measuring degrees of hardship and suffering, one cannot eliminate this appearance of vagueness and imprecision from the criterion. One who employs the criterion is not thereby absolved

---

[1]   Sacred Congregation for the Doctrine of the Faith, *Declaration on Euthanasia* (1980): ". . . is it necessary in all circumstances to have recourse to all possible remedies? In the past, moralists replied that one is never obliged to use 'extraordinary' means. This reply, which as a principle still holds good, is perhaps less clear today, by reason of the imprecision of the term and the rapid progress made in the treatment of sickness. In any case, it will be possible to make a correct judgment as to the means by studying the type of treatment to be used, its degree of complexity or risk, its cost and the possibilities of using it, and comparing these elements with the result that can be expected, taking into account the state of the sick person and his or her physical and moral resources."

from the responsibility of doing some serious thinking about the case confronting him.

The problem of difficult cases

Although the distinction between ordinary and extraordinary means is easy to state, it is not always easy to apply, because it is often not immediately apparent whether a hardship entailed by a proposed treatment would be too great to justify the treatment, or whether, likewise, the benefit promised by the treatment would be sufficiently great to justify it. Since there are no precise methods for calculating degrees of hardship or of benefit, there are inevitably borderline cases in which it may seem impossible to determine whether a given means of treatment is ordinary or extraordinary.

The difficulty of these problems is well illustrated by two features of the case of Karen Quinlan, the young American woman who suffered irreversible brain damage in 1974, after she had taken both drugs and alcohol at a party, and then remained alive but in a comatose condition for another ten years. The first point to notice is that Miss Quinlan's parents, guided by the advice of priests and physicians, recognized that their daughter's condition was hopeless, and that the artificial respiration which she was undergoing was doing no more than maintain her in a comatose state. They therefore applied to the courts for permission to have the respirator disconnected, and their request was granted. Clearly they, and those advising them, believed the artificial respiration to be an extraordinary means of preserving life. (There are surely good grounds for this belief, first because artificial respiration imposes severe burdens on many people – on relations and health professionals, if not on a comatose patient – and strains resources which could be used in other ways; and secondly because in the case of Miss Quinlan the benefit to be gained from continuing the treatment, namely, an indefinite existence in a comatose state, was too meagre to make it worthwhile.) However, the nuns who operated the hospital where Miss Quinlan was a patient believed that any attempt to discontinue the treatment which was keeping her alive in this comatose state would be immoral. So, anticipating that the courts would decide in favour of the Quinlans' request for termination of treatment, they gradually weaned her off the respirator, so that by the time the machine was eventually disconnected she was able to breathe without it. The result was that instead of dying almost immediately after the withdrawal of the apparatus, as had been expected, Miss Quinlan lingered on for another ten years in this comatose state, but now breathing spontaneously, until she finally died, of acute pneumonia, in April 1985. Now it could be that the hospital's action was motivated not by any theoretical considerations about ordinary and extraordinary means, but simply by an unthinking and unreasonable commitment to preserving life at all costs. But we have to admit that the lack of absolutely precise criteria for applying such terms as "severe hardship" and "substantial benefit" means that someone intent on maintaining artificial respiration for an irreversibly comatose patient would be able to formulate *some* defence of his action – for instance, simply by appealing to the fact that continued respiration does prolong life, even if only in a comatose state.

The second important point about the Karen Quinlan case is that although artificial respiration was withdrawn from her, the hospital continued feeding her artifically: this is, of course, why Miss Quinlan lived for so long. Now, the hospital authorities would have been justified in acting in this way only if the provision of food were always an ordinary means of preserving life. Is this the case? Is it always obligatory for health professionals to feed patients, regardless of their conditions and prospects? Here we have a difficult problem which provokes sharp disagreements, even among moralists who rely on the distinction between ordinary and extraordinary means of treatment. Admittedly, the provision of food will almost always be an ordinary means of treatment, since eating is absolutely necessary for a person's maintenance in health or return to health. But it may be that artificial feeding may sometimes be non-obligatory because it either involves serious hardship, or confers no worthwhile benefit, or both. First, consider hardship. If feeding is intravenous it will involve some discomfort for the patient, and over a long period it may add considerably to the burdens imposed on him. It will, moreover, eventually lead to breakdown in the walls of veins, and this is a real physical harm to the patient. While the felt discomfort of intravenous feeding would not *by itself* be a sufficiently grave burden to warrant its discontinuation, it could well be the "last straw", the final discomfort which, coming on top of other discomforts, makes a whole programme of treatment intolerable for a patient. This consideration obviously does not apply in the Karen Quinlan case, since Miss Quinlan was comatose. But it could be argued that the burden on other people, particularly health-care workers, and on public or private resources, which is involved in continuing to feed a patient in such a condition, is unreasonably heavy – at least in view of the very small benefit which such treatment confers. This brings us to the second criterion of something's being an extraordinary means, that of lack of benefit. Would we confer a genuine benefit on a patient by keeping him going – in principle for an indefinite period – in an irreversibly comatose state? To be sure, the patient is still alive, but he can no longer exercise those capacities and abilities which make possible a pursuit of human flourishing: he cannot participate in any of the basic goods other than life, and his participation in that one good is minimal. May we conclude, then, that any attempt by others to feed such a patient indefinitely would be unjustifiable because it would not provide him with any benefit sufficiently worthwhile to justify the labour and expense involved? In support of this conclusion one could cite some remarks made by Pope Pius XII, that ordinary means of treatment are alone obligatory, because "A more strict obligation would be too burdensome for most men and would render the attainment of the higher, more important good too difficult. Life, death, all temporal activities are in fact subordinated to spiritual ends..."[1]

It is arguable that any attempt to keep alive an irreversibly comatose patient would have to be rejected as involving a neglect of the "higher, more important good" of which the Pope was speaking, namely the human person's orientation towards the knowledge and love of God. To be *too* solicitous of one's health and bodily integrity would be to treat one's body as the be-all and end-all of existence, instead of seeing it as essentially subordinated to the spiritual goals of moral integrity and fellowship with God. It could be objected that intravenous feeding does benefit the patient in that it keeps him alive, but it is hard to see how continued physical life is a benefit if it is entirely cut off from involvement in conscious mental activity; and (it is supposed) this is precisely what happens in the case of an irreversibly comatose person.

Some ethicists contend that the symbolic importance of food and drink is so great to man, and is associated so closely with his vitality and his very existence, that any tendency in the direction of discontinuing artificial feeding, even for irreversibly comatose persons, would have a coarsening effect both on health professionals and on the general public: people's

---

[1] Pope Pius XII, Allocution to Physicians, 24 November, 1957 (*Acta Apostolicae Sedis* 49 (1957), 1031–2.)

respect for human life would inevitably be undermined. Dr. Daniel Callahan, one of the best-known American medical ethicists, takes this attitude, claiming, not that withdrawing artificial feeding would be wrong *in itself*, but that its consequences for public sentiment and public morality would be deplorable. He writes:

> I see no social disaster in the offing if there remains a deep-seated revulsion at the stopping of feeding even under legitimate circumstances. No doubt some people will live on in ways beneficial neither to them nor to others. No doubt a good bit of money will be wasted indulging rationally hard-to-defend anti-starvation policies. That strikes me as a tolerable price to pay to preserve – with ample margin to spare – one of the few moral emotions that could just as easily be called a necessary social instinct.[1]

One might reply to this argument that it is not obvious that the public's reaction would be what the author predicts. Why should it be thought that people's determination to treasure the gift of life should be undermined if it became known that irreversibly comatose patients were not being fed? An objector might urge that if discontinuation of feeding is in itself morally justified, we have no grounds for fearing that it will lead to a coarsening of people's attitude towards human life. Here we have one of those disputed questions which has not been decisively resolved one way or the other, and on which moral theologians and philosophers in the natural-law tradition often take up opposing stances. It seems to me that the view that discontinuation of artificial feeding is sometimes permissible has, at least, not been shown to be wrong, but this is very much a personal opinion, which others might want to dispute. The issue here is one on which debate is continuing and for which no "agreed position" is available.

Debilitated elderly patients: the argument resumed

We may now return to consider the issue on which discussion was postponed at the end of the last chapter, that of whether one is always obliged to to treat a debilitated elderly patient who contracts an infection such as pneumonia. Are doctors required to prescribe antibiotics to clear up the infection, or may they stand back and let nature take its course? A

---

[1]   D. Callahan, "On Feeding the Dying", *The Hastings Center Report*, vol. 13, October 1983, p. 22.

great deal depends here on the degree of debilitation from which the patient is suffering, but it is assumed that the patient is seriously debilitated, that even before the onset of the pneumonia he is subject to much mental and physical suffering and impairment, even though not obviously on the point of death. What is to be done in this sort of case?

It is evident that a doctor may not decide to withhold antibiotics from such a patient as a means of deliberately bringing about the patient's death; he may not, that is, proceed by first deciding that it would be better if the patient were to die and then working towards that end by issuing the order "No antibiotics". If he is to act rightly in withholding the drugs, he must direct his action not to bringing about the patient's death, but rather to sparing the patient avoidable suffering which would result from treatment and/or to avoiding interventions which would not genuinely benefit him. In other words, a decision not to intervene will be justified only if the antibiotics can reasonably be seen as extraordinary means of preserving the patient's life. Now, unless the patient is already taking other drugs which would be incompatible with the antibiotics, we can hardly say that administering the latter would cause him any great hardship. If, then, the antibiotics are to count as extraordinary means it will be because they offer no appreciable benefit to the patient. Is this the case or not? Here we sail upon dangerous waters, because a decision that the patient would not benefit from the antibiotics could be based on certain improper "quality-of-life" considerations. That is, someone making this decision could be reasoning as follows: "Patient X is now in such a debilitated condition that he can neither think coherently nor engage in intelligible conversation with other people. His life is therefore meaningless, devoid of value; so we are not justified in striving to keep that life going". Because the intimate details of a person's mental and spiritual life are known only to God, this kind of judgment – that someone's life is meaningless or totally worthless – is not one which human beings can ever be competent to make. We cannot, therefore, employ this line of reasoning to justify a decision not to treat. Could a doctor rightly decide on *other* grounds that antibiotic treatment should not be given?

The answer is, I think, Yes – sometimes, at least. Clearly much will depend on the degree of debilitation from which the patient is suffering, so here as with other applications of the criterion of extraordinary means, no very precise guidelines can be laid down. But it does seem that in the case of very severely debilitated patients little of benefit will be achieved by any attempt to cure the acute condition. For a patient suffering this grave debilitation has, like the irreversibly comatose patient, lost the ability to exercise those capacities which make possible a pursuit and promotion of his own flourishing; he can still participate in the basic good of life and perhaps in some of the other goods, but only to a minimal degree. By being given antibiotic treatment he may be enabled to overcome an infection, but the effect on him of the fight against the infection may be an even more severe state of debilitation. There is also the fact that death for such a patient is likely to occur in a reasonably short period of time whatever happens, and moreover that there is likely to be a recurrence of infections of the same type which will be more and more severe in their effect. In this sense any aggressive treatment of the infection is likely to be futile. It seems, then, that a doctor may sometimes reasonably decide that further aggressive treatment of an acute condition would be ill-advised. As one geriatrician has commented:

> Medical treatment must be tailored to the special features of long-stay patients. When patients are slowly and inevitably deteriorating it is essential to temper excessive therapeutic zeal. Thus resuscitation rarely has a place and in many instances it may be more fitting to withhold antibiotics for pneumonia, the old man's friend, when this ushers in a peaceful release from a long and trying illness. Quality of life and not its length should be the prime concern, and symptomatic treatment, for example with opiates for pain, should not be denied when the patient's life would be made more bearable even at the cost of some risk to its duration.[1]

The only statement in this passage to which we might demur is: "Quality of life. . . should be the prime concern". For the phrase "quality of life" can be used in such a way as to suggest that some people's lives are worthless and therefore that we should act with a view to bringing about their death. On the other hand, this is not necessarily the way in which the author of the quoted passage is using the phrase "quality of life". His statement that "Quality of life. . . should be the prime concern" may, in fact, amount to saying "we should concern ourselves above all with the extent to which we can genuinely benefit the patient". If this is what his remark amounts to, it is clearly justified. However, the words "quality of

---

[1.] H. M. Hodkinson, *An Outline of Geriatrics* (London, 1975), p. 60.

life" are capable of bearing two different senses, one of which naturally goes along with morally unacceptable judgments. We should be wise, then, not to talk at all about the quality of people's lives, but instead to think always in terms of the benefit or lack of benefit which a given course of treatment may afford.

Treatment of the terminally ill and fatally injured

The terminally ill are those who are in the final stage of an illness which will soon result in their deaths; the fatally injured, on the other hand, are those who have suffered bodily injury, usually as a result of an accident of some sort, which is so severe as to be incompatible with continued life. Despite the obvious difference between these two sorts of condition, the fact that they both have to do with the threat of imminent death means that the ethical problems which arise in treating patients belonging to these two groups are largely similar. There are, in fact, two moral difficulties which arise especially frequently with patients of both these sorts: first, the problem of whether health professionals are obliged to resuscitate a terminally-ill or fatally-injured patient if he suffers cardiac arrest; and secondly, the problem of whether one is obliged to provide these patients with artificial life support if this is necessary to keep them alive. Both these problems can, I believe, be discussed and clarified in a fairly straightforward way; but there is a third problem which is less easily handled. This is the problem of the legitimacy of organ transplantation as it is currently practised. What makes this problem particularly intractable is that in order to solve it we must first answer certain other difficult questions, such as: "How should death be defined?" and "How can we be sure that a patient is in fact dead, so that a surgical team can proceed to remove his organs for transplantation in someone else?" Because the whole issue of organ transplantation is complex and controversial, the remarks made here will inevitably be sketchy; but since the ethical problems which this practice raises are very much problems for nurses, they deserve to be given some discussion here.

(i) *Resuscitation.* Suppose that a patient in hospital has entered what are probably the final stages of his illness; death is likely within days or weeks, as far as one can tell. If this patient suffers a cardiac arrest, is the medical and nursing team obliged to try to resuscitate the patient, or could they rightly decide against it?

The team will be morally obliged to resuscitate the patient only if resuscitation can reasonably be seen as an ordinary means of treatment; if it is extraordinary there will be no obligation to resuscitate. If resuscitation is to count as an ordinary means, it must both promise some real benefit to the patient and be free of unreasonably severe hardships for him and others. Now it is certainly doubtful whether this is indeed so in the case which we are considering. For the patient is very close to the end of his life, and by resuscitating him the nurses could provide him with only a short extension of the time available to him. Sometimes this short extension may be extremely valuable, but if, for instance, the patient is under continuous sedation or has largely lost the use of those physical and mental capacities which are most typically human, it is even more questionable whether the brief extension of life which resuscitation would be a real benefit. Then again, resuscitation is often a highly painful procedure; and the pain and discomfort that it involves counts as a genuine hardship for him. If resuscitation has to be performed several times the hardship to the patient is, naturally, much greater than if it is performed only once. Nurses have often felt appalled by the sheer amount of suffering which successive resuscitations have inflicted on their patients, as in this report by a student nurse at a London hospital:

"The patient, a woman, was on a ventilator and was unconscious. She had arrested five times before I came on duty on the night shift, and then 18 more times during the night. We were told to keep resuscitation going because the coroner couldn't be contacted to advise on switching off the ventilator until the morning. I believed that this was wrong and that it was putting the nurses on duty under extreme pressure. We all felt that the best thing to do was to let the patient go peacefully."

It is reasonable to say here that where we have a patient who is close to death and for whom a brief extra period of life would (as a result of physical and mental degeneration) not count as any genuine benefit, the pain and discomfort involved in resuscitation would make that treatment an extraordinary means. Sometimes, indeed, it will be arguable that resuscitation would be not merely extraordinary and therefore optional, but positively wrong on account of the suffering which it would cause to the patient. All this presupposes that the patient has already put his spiritual and material affairs in order, in preparation for death; if this is not the case, there will, evidently, be grounds for regarding resuscitation as providing a substantial benefit for him and therefore as an ordinary (that is, obligatory) means of treatment.

(2) *The provision of artificial life-support.* The problems which we encounter when considering artificial life-support for the terminally ill and fatally injured are similar to those concerning resuscitation. Once again, it is the criterion of extraordinary means which is crucial. Does the provision or the continuation of artificial life-support constitute an ordinary or an extraordinary means? As usual, the answer must be that artificial life-support is in itself neither ordinary nor extraordinary, but will be one or the other depending on the condition of each individual patient. There will be situations in which one would reasonably judge artificial life-support to be an extraordinary and therefore dispensable means, either (i) because it would confer no real benefit on the patient, or (ii) because the discomfort which it involves would be an unreasonable hardship for him. In addition, considerations of resource allocation could be important here: even if patient A's being kept on a ventilator is not a great hardship for patient A himself, the fact that his use of the ventilator would mean its being denied to patient B, who, perhaps, would be benefited more by using it, may suffice to make it an extraordinary treatment for patient A. Indeed, it is arguable that in the latter case, one would be obliged to use the ventilator for patient B, precisely because he would derive greater benefit from it.

(iii) *Organ transplantation.* The transplantation of organs may qualify as a life-and-death matter in either or both of two ways. First, from the point of view of the recipient of an organ: if he is not given someone else's heart (or heart-and-lungs or kidneys, etc.) he will not survive once artificial life support is withdrawn. Secondly, from the point of view of the donor of the organ. If the act of removing the organ from the donor is to be justified, the surgical team must be certain that he is already dead; for if he were still alive, the surgical removal of the organ would be a homicidal act. Some organs (particularly heart, lungs and liver) need to be obtained from a donor whose heart is still beating, whereas others, particularly the kidney and cornea, do not. If, therefore, a surgeon is to be justified in removing organs belonging to the first group, he must be certain that the patient is dead, despite the fact that his heart is still beating. Here we can see why the question of determining the criterion of death has become so pressing in recent years. Surgeons want to remove organs from donors as soon as practicable after the donors' deaths. The criterion traditionally used – cessation of all cardio-pulmonary activity – would exclude all heart, heart-and-lung and liver transplants. If these organs are to be transplanted in a way which is morally acceptable it must, then, be shown that this traditional criterion of death can be overthrown in favour of one which allows that a beating-heart donor may be dead.

Ethical problems raised by organ transplantation are complex and difficult, and the following brief remarks will inevitably leave much unsaid. I shall be more interested in setting out general principles which can be applied to particular cases than in discussing particular cases themselves. And I shall consider the morality of organ transplantation in itself, neglecting other criticisms which might be made. (For instance, the objection that organ transplantation, as a high-technology and therefore extremely expensive business, wastes resources which would more bene-ficially be directed to more everyday aspects of health care, is *prima facie* a strong one. But the issues here are, once again, complex: not all trans-plantation could be objected to on grounds of resource-allocation, since kidney transplantation (for example) is a more cost-effective procedure than renal dialysis.)

First, then, consider organ transplantation from the point of view of the recipient. Is it justifiable to keep someone alive by providing him with organs taken from someone else? Clearly it is: given that the patient's life can be maintained, in the long run, only by this means, and that to maintain his life is definitely to benefit him, there is no reasonable objection to treating him in this way. The fact that the patient is receiving a bodily organ taken from someone else does not appear to raise any ethical difficulty: if the immunological problems of grafting tissues from one person's body into another can be overcome, there is no good reason not to proceed.

The one sort of case in which organ transplantation would seem morally objectionable from the recipient's point of view is that in which it is an experimental procedure without any foreseeable benefit to the recipient. Consider the case, now notorious, of Dr. Leonard Bailey's operation on a fortnight-old baby girl in October, 1984, at a surgical centre in California. Dr. Bailey transplanted the heart of a baboon into this child, who died a week later. Dr. Bailey and his team foresaw with absolute certainty that the transplant was not going to succeed and that the child – "Baby Fae", as she was called – would not last for more than a few days before the new heart was rejected by her immune system. The procedure was carried out not in order to benefit Baby Fae but as an experiment designed to improve methods and techniques of transplantation. We have here a clearly immoral procedure, involving the treatment of a child as an object to be used in the interests of medical science.

Now let us consider organ transplantation from the point of view of the donor. There are two important ethical questions. First, is it right in principle to remove organs from a dead body?; and secondly, how do we tell that a person is in fact dead, so that (provided we have answered the first question in the affirmative) we can proceed with the surgery? Concerning the first question, the answer was indicated by Pope Pius XII in a discourse devoted specifically to considering corneal transplants, but setting out principles of much more general application. He said:

> From the moral and religious point of view, there is no objection to the removal of the cornea from a corpse... [when one considers that practice in itself]. For the person who receives [the corneas], that is to say, the patient, they represent a restoration and a correction of a defect, suffered from birth or brought on by an accident. As to the corpse from which the cornea is taken, nothing is done to affect either goods to which he has a right or his right to these goods. A corpse no longer is a subject of a right in the strict sense of the word, for it is deprived of the personality which alone can be a subject of a right. The excision is not the removal of a good. The organs of sight in reality (their presence and integrity) have no longer the character of goods in a corpse because they no longer serve it and no longer have a relation to any end.[1]

A slightly different way of expressing this point is as follows. Provided that a person has given permission, during his lifetime, for his bodily organs to be donated to someone else, there can be no objection to a surgeon's removing them. For a dead body is no longer a person but rather the remains of a person. Christians who accept that a human person is constituted by a human soul as well as physical matter believe that it is the soul which, by its presence, makes the matter which it "in-forms" to be a human body. What happens at death is that although the spiritual soul continues to exist it no longer animates or "in-forms" the matter to

---

[1] Pope Pius XII, Discourse to specialists in eye surgery, 14 May, 1956, quoted from *The Human Body: Papal Teachings*, selected and arranged by the Monks of Solesmes, p. 381.

which it was formerly united. A corpse is, then, not a person but the remains of a person; it should not even be called "a human body" any more, but rather the remains of a human body. It no longer functions in a recognizably human way to fulfil the goals and activities which are characteristic of human beings. Hence in removing an organ from a corpse a surgeon does not in any way attack the basic goods of a human person, precisely because there is no human person there. In principle, then, there can be no objection to removing organs from a dead body. It is normally accepted that since such action involves interfering with matter which used to constitute the body of a human person, the surgeon should previously have obtained that person's permission during his lifetime. But provided that this permission has been given, there is no objection to his acting in this way.

The real difficulty is that of establishing that death has occurred. Nowadays it is commonly believed that the brain, as the organ or set of organs which controls the operations of all the other bodily organs, is crucially important. On this view, if the workings of the brain, or some strategically important part of the brain, breaks down completely and irreversibly, the failure of all the other vital functions will inevitably follow. This argument does not show that death of the brain *is* the death of the whole body, but rather that the one event leads to the other within a short time. But many people would claim that brain death is a sufficient indication of the absence of human life or personhood even if the body still displays some residual powers. For, it is argued, the brain is that organ which "underlies" and makes possible the mental activities of thinking, deliberating, willing and so on which are characteristic of human beings. If, then, the appropriate brain functioning is impossible, these mental activities cannot take place, and hence the body which one is treating is no longer the body of a person; it is a "mere" body and can be treated as such.[1]

[1.] Dr. Christopher Pallis, the leading British proponent of brain-stem death as a criterion of death of the whole person, defines death as

... a state in which there is irreversible loss of the capacity for consciousness combined with irreversible loss of the capacity to breathe (and hence to maintain a heart beat). Alone, neither would be sufficient. Both are essentially brain stem functions (predominantly represented, incidentally, at different ends of the brain stem)... Although seldom explicitly formulated, this view of death is, I believe, widely shared in the West. It is the implicit basis for British practice in diagnosing "brain death". (C. Pallis, *ABC of Brain Stem Death* (London, 1983), p. 2.)

Nowadays the criterion standardly used to detect death is not that of the death of the brain as a whole – this would be too difficult to ascertain, even with the aid of electroencephalographic tests – but rather that of the brain stem.[1] For the brain stem controls the body's capacity to breathe and hence to maintain a spontaneous heartbeat. If the brain stem dies, cessation of the heartbeat follows soon afterwards; even if ventilation is maintained artificially, the heart is able to continue beating spontaneously for only a period of between 48 and 72 hours.[2] Moreover, a functioning brain stem is required also for conscious awareness and the proper functioning of the cerebral hemispheres. Hence, it is argued, it is reasonable to identify the death of the brain stem with the death of the whole person. This will be true even when the other parts of the brain, and in particular the two cortical hemispheres, are still functioning to some extent. It is, then, arguable that "all death is indeed brainstem death, and that one only dies. . . because one's brainstem has ceased to function", and hence that death "is, and always has been, brainstem death".[3]

This argument has achieved a wide currency, but it is disputable whether personhood and brain functioning are related as closely as its supporters claim. If we accept the traditional Christian view that there is a spiritual soul in man which, together with the matter making up his body, constitutes him as the sort of psycho-physical being which he is, there will be some doubt about the closeness of the connexion between the continued existence of an embodied human being and the continuance of brain functioning. Many people today – including, probably, most neurophysiologists and philosophers who study these matters – think of human mental activity as impossible without the functioning of a brain, but all that has definitely been established is that damage to the brain normally results in impairment and distortion of our mental activities. It has not been shown that what happens under normal conditions in an embodied human person must always happen, or that there could not be mental activity in the total absence of any functioning brain. The sort of

---

[1] In the United States the criterion used is often that of a flat EEG scan, which indicates an absence of neural activity in the cerebral cortex. However, a flat EEG scan is quite compatible with the continued occurrence of neural activity in the brain stem. It does not, therefore, necessarily indicate that the brain as a whole is dead. (See R. E. Barry, O.P., "Ethics and Brain Death", in *The New Scholasticism*, vol. 61, no. 1, 1987, pp. 82–98.)

[2] See C. Pallis, "Brain Stem Death – The Evolution of a Concept", in *The Medico-Legal Journal*, vol. 55, 1987, Part Two, pp. 84–107, at p. 96.

[3] Pallis, "Brain Stem Death – The Evolution of a Concept", p. 97.

position maintained by the French philosopher Henri Bergson (1859–1941), that the central nervous system is essentially directed to the selection and preparation of overt bodily behaviour, and that there is no detailed correspondence between brain activity and mental activity, is still, it seems to me, a live philosophical option.[1] More generally, it is arguable that the soul remains present in the body for as long as the latter displays any of the vital signs of life, such as cardiac and respiratory activity. Admittedly, some authors who accept the view that man is a composite of spiritual soul and matter have also defended the brain-death criterion, but it has been shown that there is some doubt about the consistency of holding these two positions together.[2] So the brain-death criterion of the death of a person appears to be unsatisfactory. The only safe course of action for a surgical team wishing to transplant organs is, it seems, to rely on the traditional criterion of death in terms of the complete cessation of all vital signs, including cardio-pulmonary activity. If reliance on this more conservative criterion should render some transplant operations more difficult or even impossible to carry out, this is something we should be obliged to put up with: to favour the brain-death criterion simply because it would facilitate one's surgical aims would be to favour doing evil so that good might come. Where does this leave a nurse who is supposed to take part in the transplantation of a vital organ? If the surgeon intends to rely on the brain-death criterion to establish that the donor is dead he will act wrongly in proceeding with the operation. The nurse who co-operates formally with him will also, then, act wrongly.

This is about as much as we can usefully say about these difficult problems without grossly exceeding the compass of this book. Two points, in particular, should be noted: first, the vital importance of the distinction

---

1. Cf. H. Bergson, *Matter and Memory*, trans. N.M. Paul and W. Scott Palmer (London, 1913) and also Bergson's essay "The Soul and the Body", in his *Mind-Energy*, trans. H. Wildon Carr (London, 1920), pp. 29–59. A more recent defence of a similar thesis can be found in K. R. Popper and J. C. Eccles, *The Self and its Brain* (Berlin, 1977).

2. For an argument that the brain-death criterion is incompatible with any belief in a spiritual soul as constituting the nature of man, see Mary R. Hayden, "A Philosophical Critique of the Brain Death Movement", *Linacre Quarterly*, vol. 49, August, 1982, pp. 240–247.

between ordinary and extraordinary means in dealing with the problems surveyed here; and secondly, the fact that this principle is not one which can be applied in a mechanical and unthinking manner. Here as elsewhere, the recognition of the truth of moral principles certainly does not do away with the need to do some hard thinking about their mode of application.

★　★　★

This Chapter in Summary

Moralists in the natural-law tradition, faced with questions of the form "Are we obliged to try to keep this patient alive or not?", have relied on the distinction between ordinary and extraordinary means. This distinction is widely misunderstood, because it is not realized (1) that the words "ordinary" and "extraordinary" are being used in a special technical sense, and (2) that whether or not some means of treatment is an extraordinary means is dependent on the particular condition and circumstances of each individual patient, so that one and the same treatment may be ordinary for patient A but extraordinary for patient B (or for patient A at a different stage in his life). Using this principle we can go some way, at least, towards resolving problems concerning resuscitation and the treatment of debilitated elderly patients. However, there are certain other problems, especially those concerning artificial feeding of irreversibly comatose patients, which seem recalcitrant to any cut-and-dried solution. Concerning organ transplantation, while there is no strong objection to the practice in itself, any attempt to base transplantation procedures on the brain-stem criterion of death would seem to be objectionable, since the idea that a person whose brain stem has ceased to function is dead is open to grave doubt.

CHAPTER TWELVE

PROBLEMS OF LIFE AND DEATH – (3)

Two key principles – the principle of double effect and the principle that extraordinary means of preserving life are not morally obligatory – have figured prominently in the discussion so far of life-and-death issues. In this chapter we shall see that these principles are relevant also to the two kinds of problem which now require to be considered: abortion and the treatment of the handicapped new-born.

Abortion

The practice of abortion raises two important moral issues for nurses. First, is abortion ever justified? Secondly, if abortion is (usually or even always) an immoral deed, may a nurse nevertheless, under some circumstances and to some extent, co-operate with those performing abortions? If so, precisely under what sorts of circumstances, and to what extent? When (if at all) would co-operation be absolutely wrong?

For a nurse working in a British hospital, the problem of abortion will often assume the form of the question: "Should I declare myself a conscientious objector to abortion so as to be able to 'opt out' of participating in terminations?" For Section Four the 1967 Abortion Act gives doctors and nurses the right to take this step. If a nurse decides that abortion is always morally wrong she may declare to the hospital authorities that she believes it to be wrong and wishes to have no part in any such operations. The principal issue here is, then, whether she should conclude that abortion is intrinsically immoral. Are there grounds for holding this?

Catholic moral philosophers and theologians have traditionally asserted that abortion is, like murder or suicide or adultery, one of those acts which are wrong *of their very nature*. On this view an act of abortion is wrong as such and always, regardless of what the consequences of either aborting or not aborting might happen to be. In recent times this total rejection of abortion has been expressed vigorously by Pope Pius XII (d. 1958):

> As long as a man is not guilty, his life is untouchable, and therefore any act directly tending to destroy it is illicit, whether such destruction is intended as an end in itself or only as a means to an end,

whether it is a question of life in the embryonic stage or in a stage of final development or already in its final stages.[1]

In 1965, the Second Vatican Council declared: "Life must be safeguarded with extreme care from conception; abortion and infanticide are abominable crimes."[2] And this rejection of abortion, not just in certain special circumstances but unconditionally, was reiterated in the *Declaration on Procured Abortion*, issued by the Vatican in 1974. This declaration states, in part:

> Respect for human life is called for from the time that the process of generation begins. From the time that the ovum is fertilized, a life is begun which is neither that of the father nor of the mother; it is rather the life of a new human being with its own growth. It would never be made human if it were not human already.[3]

This condemnation of abortion explicitly presupposes that what happens in abortion is that a human foetus, which is a living human being, is deliberately killed. So what is being condemned is the deliberate killing of the foetus, not the act of tolerating its death as the side-effect of (say) certain other measures directed towards saving its mother's life. It is claimed that this act of killing, like other killings of innocent human beings, cannot be justified under any circumstances. The argument, in other words, is as follows:

(1) The foetus is an innocent human being in the full sense of the words "human being", that is, a human person.

(2) Intentionally to kill an innocent human being is always wrong, and this holds whatever might be the consequences of killing or not killing.

(3) In abortion, what happens is precisely that a human foetus is intentionally killed.

---

[1]   Pope Pius XII, Allocution to the Medical-Biological Union of St. Luke (1944), translated in *The Human Body: Papal Teachings*, selected and arranged by the monks of Solesmes (Boston, U.S.A., 1979), p. 60.

[2]   *Gaudium et Spes* (Pastoral Constitution on the Church in the Modern World), section 51.

[3]   Sacred Congregation for the Doctrine of the Faith, *Declaration on Procured Abortion*, in A. Flannery (ed.), *Vatican Council II: More Postconciliar Documents* (Leominster, 1982), p. 445. For a comprehensive historical study of the Catholic Church's attitude to abortion, see J. R. Connery, *Abortion: The Development of the Roman Catholic Perspective* (Chicago, 1977).

Therefore:

> (4) Abortion as such is wrong – it is wrong always and everywhere, regardless of any considerations about consequences.

This argument is clearly valid; that is, if all three premises are true the conclusion must be true also. Now premise (3) is true simply by definition, because abortion just is the deliberate killing of a human foetus. The absolute prohibition of abortion, therefore, depends crucially upon premises (1) and (2). Premise (2) is, in fact, a statement of the principle that it is wrong to kill an innocent human being. Someone favouring abortion may reject this moral principle and argue that deliberate killing is justifiable whenever it would be productive of great good. But he would have to apply this principle consistently, not only to abortion but also to the sorts of cases examined in Chapter Six (destructive experimentation on children; killing someone who has made a will in one's favour; and so on). But the immorality of these acts is surely so obvious that most pro-abortionists would shrink from applying the principle across the board and would thus be guilty of inconsistency. I suspect that most pro-abortionists would admit that the killing of innocent human beings is always and in principle wrong, while adding: "But the foetus isn't a human being!"

This brings us to premise (1). Someone attacking this premise would want to say that the human foetus is not a human being in the full sense; that is, that it is not yet *a human person* but rather becomes a person at some later stage – this stage being after conception and, probably, prior to birth, but otherwise not identifiable with any great precision. The foetus, he would add, is evidently a human being in the sense that it is composed of organic material which is recognizably human rather than feline or canine or equine, etc. – it normally has 46 chromosomes and is destined to develop into a mature human being if nothing prevents it from doing so – but to say this is certainly not to say that it is already a human person. Suppose that a woman has undergone a laparoscopy, perhaps as part of an *in vitro* fertilization programme, so that several of her ova are now lying in a petri dish in a medical laboratory. These ova are, in a sense, "human beings", because their genetic constitution marks them out as specifically human tissue. Also, they could be said to be *potentially* human persons, because if they were to be united with male spermatozoa and allowed to develop in the appropriate environment, they would eventually become fully-fledged persons capable of thinking, feeling, deliberating and making choices, having emotions, conversing with others, and so on. But these ova are not actually, here and now, human beings in the full sense, that is, human persons. For at present they can perform none of those typically human activities just listed, and this range of activities is the criterion by which alone we judge something to be a person or not. Moreover, what holds of sperm and ovum taken separately holds also of the human embryo and foetus, which also fail to measure up to the criteria of full personhood. So, it is concluded, since foetuses are not persons they cannot have the rights which we accord to persons, and in particular they lack the right to life; we may therefore destroy them through abortion if we have good reason to do so.[1]

Evidently the crux of the argument between the pro- and anti-abortionist is this question of whether or not the foetus is a human being in the full sense of those words, that is, a *person*. The pro-abortionist answers in the negative because the foetus does not perform any of those conscious mental activities which we ordinarily regard as typical of persons. This type of argument will apply even more obviously to the human embryo which is only a few hours or days old than to a foetus of (say) three months. For whereas the foetus will, at that stage, be recognizably human and have most of its organs developed and functioning, the embryo does not even look specifically human: to all appearances it is nothing more than a roughly circular collection of cells, with no coherent structure and no distinguishable parts with specialized functions. (This is not, of course, the case. The embryo possesses a clear developmental structure which accounts for its progressive growth as a single organism. But the point is that this developmental structure is by no means obvious "on the surface".) Someone who favours scientific experimentation on human embryos is therefore likely to appeal to the same kind of argument as that of the pro-abortionist.

[1.]   This argument, that the foetus (or, at least, the early embryo) is "a potential being" in the same sense as are the male and female gametes taken separately, and therefore deserves no greater protection than they do, is commonly employed nowadays. See, e.g., The Warnock Report (official title: *Report of the Committee of Inquiry into Human Fertilisation and Embryology*) (London, 1984), section 11.9, p. 60; and P. Singer and D. Wells, *The Reproduction Revolution* (Oxford, 1984), who state (pp. 90–91): "[the human embryo] has the potential to develop into a normal human being, with a high degree of rationality, self-consciousness, autonomy and so on. Can this potential justify the belief that the embryo is entitled to a special moral status? We believe that it cannot, for the following reason. Everything that can be said about the potential of the embryo can also be said about the potential of the egg and sperm when separate but considered jointly."

The status of the human foetus

A pro-abortionist may regard the argument sketched above as completely decisive. But the argument is, in fact, based on a misconception of the criteria which we normally employ for affirming that someone is a person. For, admittedly, the concept of a person is closely connected with the idea of certain important mental capacities, such as the capacities to think and reason, to deliberate over courses of action and make choices, and to engage in conversation with other people. It is precisely because we believe that all the animals lower than man lack these capacities that we deny them the status of persons. But here we must be clear about just what we mean by the word "capacity". The pro-abortionist evidently means to deny that unborn children and human embryos have the capacity to think, to deliberate and choose, etc.; but the truth of this denial is by no means beyond doubt, because it can be maintained that unborn children – and even a day-old or hour-old embryo – do have all these capacities, and therefore deserve to be recognized as persons.

Here we need to distinguish between two ways of understanding the term "capacity" or "potentiality". This distinction can be illustrated by some simple examples. Suppose we say of a schoolboy that he has a certain capacity, such as the capacity to play the trumpet or to speak in German. We may mean that the boy has already learnt to perform the activity in question, so that if he is handed a trumpet he can immediately play something, or if he is asked a question in German he can respond to it intelligently in that language. So, on this understanding of the word "capacity", someone has a capacity to do X if, having chosen to do X, and providing that external conditions in no way inhibit him from acting, he is able here and now to do X. But there is another sense of the word "capacity" in which someone who has not learnt to do X and so could not do X at a moment's notice, even if he chose to, nevertheless does have the capacity to do X. A six-month-old baby cannot play the trumpet or speak any language at all, but it still makes perfectly good sense to say that he has the capacity to play the trumpet, or to speak in German, or to dance a quick-step. For although he cannot at the moment actually do any of these things, he does possess the ability to learn to do them. This ability can be brought to fruition only over a period of time, but it is present here and now in the six-month-old child. We must therefore distinguish between a capacity as a *present ability*, that is, an ability possessed here and now to act in a certain way, and what we might call a *radical capacity*, an ability rooted in one's nature by which one comes eventually, and as a result of experience and training, to have capacities in the first sense, that is, present abilities.

We must, therefore, distinguish between: first, the actual performance of some activity; secondly, the possession of a present ability to perform the activity; and thirdly, the possession of a radical capacity to come to perform it. Suppose that Mrs. White is a fluent speaker of German. If she is not at this moment speaking in German, she is not actually exercising her present ability to do so, but that present ability remains a real feature of her, one of her intrinsic attributes. Even if Mrs. White is sound asleep, her ability to speak German is a real characteristic which remains in her, and which she may actually exercise when she wakes up; whereas her husband, who (let us suppose) is a typically monolingual Englishman, does not have this real characteristic. There is, then, a real difference between Mr. and Mrs. White which persists through time, even when Mrs. White is not actually exercising her knowledge of German. However, although Mr. White is neither speaking German now nor in possession of the present ability to do so, he does have the *radical capacity* to do so, because he can work through a manual of German grammar, or attend evening classes, and as a result acquire a working knowledge of the language. This radical capacity is a real feature of Mr. White, just as real a feature of him as the corresponding present ability is of his wife. We see this if we contrast Mr. White with his pet canary, who has no such radical capacity: one may enrol the canary at the Goethe Institut and subject the hapless bird to any amount of instruction, but it will never come to understand spoken German or to converse in it. The difference between Mr. White and his pet is, then, a difference of nature; Mr. White's radical capacity to come to speak German is a real characteristic of him, a real feature of *what he is*, which the canary lacks.

To return to the debate over abortion, the pro-abortionist's argument is that a human foetus, since it cannot think or deliberate or choose, etc., is not a person; for unless something has these higher mental abilities we do not count it as a person. But in arguing thus he overlooks the crucial distinction between a present ability and a radical capacity of human nature. For while the foetus does not possess any of the present abilities to act in those ways which are characteristically human, he does possess the radical capacities which, in time and after the appropriate training and stimulus, will result in his having all those present abilities. His present possession of these radical capacities sets him apart from all other bodily creatures, because the capacities are real characteristics which he has right from the beginning of his existence but which they lack. The reply could be made that the radical capacities in question are not present right from the beginning of the foetus's existence but somehow supervene on it later on in life – so that only at that later point does it become a human being in the full sense. There seems no way of decisively refuting this option, but all the evidence is against it. For the physical constitution of a human being is laid down once and for all at fertilization, its subsequent history being a matter of the unfolding and developing of its potentialities. Before that point, we have not one individual organism but two – a male spermatozoon and a female ovum – neither of which, by itself, possesses any inherent capability of growth and development. But once the ovum has been fertilized, we have an entirely new single being which is some-thing over and above the two gametes which combined to produce it: it is a new kind of being, with a new nature. The proof of this is that if the embryo is provided with food and the right environment, it has the wherewithal (unlike the sperm and ovum taken separately) to grow eventually into a fully mature member of the species *homo sapiens*. There is present in the foetus, and indeed in the human embryo, a sort of inner orientation to the mature specimen which it will (all being well) some day become. Given that the history of the foetus subsequent to fertilization is one of continuous development, with no abrupt changes of direction which might indicate the sudden acquisition of new capacities or characteristics, it is reasonable to suppose that all the radical capacities for engaging in characteristically human activities are present in the embryo as soon as fertilization has been completed. What we have after fertiliza-tion, then, is a human being in the full sense, a human person. It is not true that the embryo or foetus is "a potential human being". Such talk seems appropriate only because people are inclined to confuse the notion of potentiality with that of *immaturity*. The embryo or foetus is a human being in a markedly immature state, because all the radical capacities of human nature which are present in it have barely begun to be developed; but it nevertheless now possesses all these capacities, and this is what matters as far as our right to call it "a human being" or "a human person" is concerned. A one-year-old child is an immature specimen of humanity (although much less so than a week-old embryo) and has practically the whole of the unfolding and maturation of his natural capacities in front of him, but we could not, on this account, call him "a potential human being". He is every bit as much an actual human being as is a 40-year-old man, the difference between them being that the 40-year-old is a mature specimen – his natural capacities have been largely actualized and brought to fruition – whereas the one-year-old is at a much earlier stage of maturation.[1] Only by carelessly conflating these distinct notions of potentiality and immaturity could someone claim that human embryos and foetuses are not human beings in the full sense but only "potential human beings".[2]

Abortion, infanticide and other deliberate killings

The argument against abortion which is being employed here presupposes that the decisive criterion for counting something a human person is possession of the radical capacities for acquiring the present abilities to think, choose, etc. Since we have every reason to believe that the human embryo and foetus possess all these radical capacities, we are bound to

---

[1] It is remarkable how those who wish to promote legalized abortion, or experimentation on human embryos, persist in describing the embryo or foetus as "a potential human being" and in ignoring the argument to the contrary. So we find the Warnock Committee stating what they take to be the argument against embryo experimentation in the following terms: "The human embryo is seen as having the same status as a child or an adult, by virtue of its potential for human life". But the opponent of experimentation will insist that the embryo is an actual person and that only someone wedded to a grossly pictorial way of conceiving things could regard it as a potential person only. Unfortunately, even the three members of the Warnock Committee who dissented from their colleagues' endorsement of experimentation (Mrs. M. Carriline, Dr. J. Marshall and Mrs. J. Walker) justified their dissent in the following terms: ". . . the embryo has a special status because of its potential for development to a stage at which everyone would accord it the status of a human person. It is in our view wrong to create something with the potential for becoming a human person and then deliberately to destroy it." (The Warnock Report, Expression of Dissent B, pp. 90–91.) The dissenters go on to make it clear that the word "potential", as it applies to the human embryo, bears a different sense from that which it has as applied to the male and female gametes. But they do not seem to suspect that this difference of meaning is so radical as to make the very use of the adjective "potential" in this context inappropriate.

[2] For Catholics and other Christians, the facts appealed to in this argument – that the genetic constitution of a man is laid down at the time of fertilization, and that his subsequent physical and mental development is continuous rather than displaying any abrupt "leap" at any stage – strongly suggest that the human soul, which constitutes any human being *as* a human being, is present right from the time of fertilization. The belief that what exists after fertilization is a human person often goes along with a belief in a spiritual soul which is created directly by God and is present in man from fertilization onwards, but the former belief can be defended without any explicit reference to, or reliance upon, doctrines concerning the soul, and this is what I have tried to do here.

conclude that a human foetus is a human person and hence that any deliberate destruction of it is as evil as a deliberate killing of a mature human being. Perhaps, however, someone could object that it is possession of the appropriate present abilities which constitutes someone a human person, not possession of the corresponding radical capacities. On this view, until a foetus's radical capacities of human nature have been actualized and developed to a reasonable degree, we cannot claim that it is a human being. What response can be made to someone arguing in this way?

Any decision to restrict the application of the word "person" to comparatively mature specimens of humanity would, I submit, be found untenable, because it would commit one to denying that many individual human beings whom we all recognize to be persons really are such. For example, new-born babies and people suffering from impaired mental functioning as a result of a stroke are surely full human beings, not merely potential ones, but they do not possess the range of present abilities which would be regarded, on the basis of this pro-abortionist move, as so decisive. Someone who adopts this line of thought should be prepared to countenance not only abortion but also infanticide. Suppose that a couple decide that they do not want their new-born baby. Would they act rightly if they have it killed? If one answers "No", it is presumably on the grounds that the baby is a human person who may not be killed; but then one is surely committed to making the same judgment concerning a three-month-old child *in utero*, because the difference between it and the neonate in terms of their present abilities for characteristically human activities is decidedly small. Conversely, if one judges that the foetus is so deficient in terms of its present abilities as not to count as a person, one must also, to be consistent, make the same judgment about a new-born baby, or indeed a one-year-old child and perhaps even older children.[1]

---

1. Professor Michael Tooley is unusual among advocates of liberal abortion laws in recognizing that acceptance of abortion commits one also to accepting infanticide. As he says, summarizing the argument of his book *Abortion and Infanticide* (Oxford, 1983): "If the line of thought pursued above is correct, neither abortion, nor infanticide, at least during the first few weeks after birth, is morally wrong. . . [for] an entity cannot be a person unless it possesses, or has previously possessed, the capacity for thought. And the psychological and neurophysiological evidence makes it most unlikely that humans, in the first few weeks after birth, possess this capacity." (Pp. 419, 421.) Clearly the human embryo or foetus lacks the capacity for thought if "capacity" is taken to be what I have called a present ability; but the radical capacity for thinking is present right from the moment of fertilization.

But surely we all recognize that the new-born baby is a human person, not just a potential human person. And in that case we must recognize that the foetus is in the same position as more mature specimens of humanity and is therefore entitled, to exactly the same extent, to protection from death-dealing attack.

The unborn child is, then, just as much a person as an adult man or woman. The only important difference between a foetus and an adult is in terms of their level of maturity: an adult is a fully mature member of the species *homo sapiens*, whereas the foetus is a member of that same species whose fundamental potentialities and capacities are largely undeveloped. But since a person's level of maturity has no bearing on his right to have his life respected – it is not, for example, a worse crime to kill a 16-year-old than a six-year-old – this fact of the immaturity of the foetus is not a ground for disposing of it through abortion. The killing of the unborn child by abortion is, then, an intrinsically wrong act, and this means that it is not to be performed whatever the consequences, that is, whatever benefits and advantages it might produce and whatever misfortunes or disasters it might enable us to avoid.

The nurse and abortion procedures

Because abortion amounts to the deliberate killing of an innocent person and is therefore wrong, nurses are obliged not to co-operate formally in abortion procedures. This means, first and foremost, that they should not participate in the actual procedure itself: they should not assist the surgeon if the procedure is a dilatation and curettage, nor should they assist in setting up a prostaglandin drip if labour is to be induced. Since the 1967 Abortion Act gives the nurse the legal right to opt out of all such procedures, she should declare herself a conscientious objector to abortion under the provisions of Section Four of that Act. Her decision to opt out should be communicated in writing to the hospital authorities as soon as she takes up her position; if she fails to do this, she could one day find herself rostered for a termination, thereby being forced to object verbally, and at short notice, to the arrangement.

A nurse who actually takes part in the procedure by which an unborn child is destroyed co-operates formally in the procedure, according to the criteria for formal co-operation which were set out in Chapter Seven: for what she actually does is specifically geared to the destruction of the foetus. Hence all such participation is morally wrong. Some other nursing procedures connected with abortion are, however, more problematic. Two such procedures call for consideration here: first, the provision of pre-medication for patients who are about to undergo terminations, and secondly, the nursing care of patients after they have had abortions. What are we to say of these activities? Do they amount to formal co-operation in abortion? If not, may they sometimes be justified?

(1) *The provision of pre-medication.* If we consider this issue carefully in the light of the appropriate moral principles concerning co-operation, the result seems to be as follows. In providing pre-medication, a nurse may not formally co-operate in the abortion; if the pre-medication amounts to material co-operation, she may provide it, but only under certain definite and restricted conditions. In particular, the co-operation must be sufficiently "remote" from the abortion itself, and the consequences of not co-operating must be sufficiently grave, either for the nurse or for others, to justify her in co-operating. Whether these conditions apply will be a matter to decide from case to case. The important question at present is: When does the provision of pre-medication amount to material co-operation only?

The answer to this question is, I believe, as follows. Pre-medication will count as material co-operation in abortion only if the nurse in no way intentionally gears her actions towards the goal of bringing about the destruction of the unborn child; and this means that to avoid co-operating formally the nurse may not provide any treatment or take any test which has the sole point of facilitating this specific procedure (*sc.*, termination of pregnancy). In other words, in caring for a patient who is to undergo a termination, she may provide only what we might call "lowest-common-denominator nursing care", that is, nursing care which would be appropriate for *any* patient of this particular age and condition of health, regardless of the nature of the treatment which she was awaiting. It will often be difficult to determine what this very general nursing care will encompass and what it will exclude, but the task is not impossible. For certain aspects of nursing care are in no way specifically orientated to abortion (e.g., keeping the patient generally comfortable; providing food; taking blood pressure, etc.) while there are others which definitely are so orientated (e.g., assisting in the setting-up of a prostaglandin drip). To perform an action of the latter sort would be to co-operate formally in the abortion, by sharing in the physician's (and the mother's) death-dealing intention; but actions of the former sort – those belonging to "lowest-common-denominator nursing care" – are not ruled out on this score.

(2) *Caring for patients after they have had abortions*. At first sight the provision of aftercare to abortion patients is unproblematic, because the deed has already been done and cannot be undone. The patient has had the abortion and nothing which a nurse may do or refuse to do can bring her child back to life. So a nurse who cares for such a patient cannot be said to facilitate her abortion; she cares for the patient and facilitates her restoration to health, but she in no way co-operates in the killing of the unborn child. Nevertheless, the fact that nursing care is all the time *available* for patients who are going to have abortions is something which enables abortions to be carried out. If such a large number of nurses were unavailable for the aftercare of abortion patients that this aftercare could not be provided, many abortions which would otherwise take place would be prevented. The nurse who provides this nursing care therefore co-operates materially with the practice of abortion in general, so she needs to justify her co-operation in some way. If she were able to opt out of aftercare for abortion patients entirely, she would have to do so. But this option is not available to her: she cannot normally pick and choose those patients whom she is prepared to care for and those whom she is not. She would be obliged to pick and choose if by doing so she could help to undermine the practice of abortion itself, thus contributing to its disappearance from her hospital or even from society at large. However, such an outcome would be possible only if there were many other nurses prepared to take the same stand, and this is not the case at present. So a nurse who contemplates the idea of withdrawing herself from the after-care of abortion patients must realize that in present circumstances her action would not affect the provision of abortion in hospitals, while on the other hand it would probably produce real harm for herself. Provided, then, that all the conditions for justified material co-operation are met – including the need to avoid giving scandal to others – it would seem that nurses would act rightly in caring for patients who have had abortions.

Advising patients who are seeking abortion

Among the possible ways of co-operating formally in an evil practice is that of advising or recommending that someone take part in such a practice. The reason for this is clear: if, for instance, Nurse A advises her patient to agree to undergo some immoral treatment X, this can only be because Nurse A has set herself the goal of having X administered to the patient; and this orientation of Nurse A's will is itself wrong. Since abortion is an evil procedure, one may not formally co-operate in bringing it about. It follows that a nurse may not advise or recommend that a patient undergo abortion. Suppose, however, that we have the following situation:

> Nurse James is a health visitor who has been helping Miss Martin, a woman with two children whose *de facto* husband abandoned her some time ago. The younger child has been having difficulties with feeding, and Nurse James has lately found herself calling regularly at Miss Martin's flat. During her latest visit, Miss Martin tells her that she is convinced that she is pregnant again, this time by another man with whom she has recently had a fleeting liaison. She doubts whether she would be able to cope with another child, and is strongly inclined to seek a termination. She asks Nurse James to tell her how she should go about obtaining one.

Nurse James, let us suppose, recognizes abortion as intrinsically wrong. She may not, then, advise or encourage Miss Martin to seek an abortion; for in doing so she would commit herself to the goal of procuring the destruction of her unborn child. How, then, should she respond to her patient's request? Should she simply refuse to give information which would facilitate Miss Martin's desire for an abortion, or should she suppress any expression of her own opinions and give her patient, in an entirely "neutral", non-judgmental way, the information she is seeking? Or should she, while informing Miss Martin of the procedure to be followed in arranging for an abortion, also express her own views on the subject, together with suggestions of ways in which Miss Martin could be supported through the pregnancy and in the period afterwards, in the hope that she might change her mind?

The first of these three options – an absolute refusal to give the information and advice requested – would seem impossible in the present climate of medical and nursing opinion. Admittedly, the code of practice under which the health visitor works may not say anything explicitly on this type of problem. Nevertheless, employing authorities would generally maintain that health visitors must give their patients information on all relevant treatments which are legally available, and that one of these treatments is termination of pregnancy. They could also regard any refusal to do this as warranting dismissal. In these circumstances it seems reasonable to regard the bare giving of information which one is required to give as an instance of material co-operation which is justifiable in view of the serious consequences which a refusal to do so could bring.

It may be, then, that the second possible course of action is correct. If it is clear that Miss Martin's mind is made up or that she would resent being advised against abortion, this option – bare presentation of the facts and nothing more – may be the sensible one to take. But suppose that Miss Martin is not absolutely determined to seek an abortion, that there is some doubt in her mind about whether she should take this step. Is Nurse James still obliged to avoid any attempt to persuade her to change her mind? The answer, I think, is clearly No: as long as Nurse James refrains from attempting to browbeat Miss Martin into a change of heart, or in any other way treating her without that respect to which she is entitled, she not only may but should attempt to enable Miss Martin to see that she is proposing something wrong. If Miss Martin proves to be unreceptive to any attempt at persuasion that will, naturally, be the end of the matter: Nurse James will be able to drop the subject, content that she has done everything in her power to save the unborn child. But as long as there is some hope of encouraging a change of mind on Miss Martin's part, Nurse James should do what she can to bring this about.

Against this, it could be argued that by acting in this way the nurse would fail to respect her patient as a free and autonomous agent and would therefore act unprofessionally. The argument would run as follows. In her work the nurse acts not as an individual, as a law unto herself, but as a health *professional*, a representative of the nursing profession. As such she is concerned not to ensure that her own personal viewpoint prevails but to uphold the standards to which the profession is committed. One of these standards is an absolute respect for the integrity of the human person as a rational and autonomous being; and this respect precludes the nurse from attempting to coerce or even to *persuade* her patient to take the course of action which she (the nurse) thinks right. The nurse is there to assist the patient, to explain to her what she needs to have explained and to enable her decisions to be put into effect; but she is not there to dictate to the patient, to decide for her what to do. Any decision on treatment or non-treatment, of whatever kind, is the patient's decision alone, and the nurse acts unprofessionally if she tries to influence her decision one way or the other.[1]

This is the argument against the idea that Nurse James should try to dissuade Miss Martin from resorting to abortion, expressed, I think, as convincingly as it can be expressed. A presupposition of the argument is that attempting to guide a patient's choice is incompatible with treating him as a free and responsible agent. But this is surely not the case: it may, in fact, be that one respects a patient precisely by refusing to leave him to his own resources and by using one's technical *and moral* knowledge to attempt to guide him. Certainly health professionals have no inhibitions about advising their patients what to do in the interests of their health ("I personally think that you have no other option – that you really must say 'Yes' to this treatment"; or, alternatively, "I think that this treatment wouldn't be justified at present, and that you would be unwise to insist on it"). Nobody would claim that a doctor or nurse who attempts to guide a patient's choice in this way would fail to respect him as an individual and would therefore act unprofessionally. Why should the situation change when the treatment is objectionable not as being physically harmful but as being morally wrong? Does "being a professional" mean that while one is on duty one must never allow one's moral convictions to influence what one says and does?

One could answer "Yes" to this question only if one were in the grip of a false conception of what a professional is and why his being a professional is important. The point of having professions in society is that they promote the genuine good of individual people and, through them, of society as a whole. And when we talk about the "genuine good" of people we must mean their *total* good, their good as whole persons. For even though the health-care professions are concerned primarily with one aspect of the human good, that of health or bodily well-functioning, doctors and nurses should not consider their patients just as bodies to be repaired or kept going as long as possible. Physical well-being is an important aspect of the human good, but human beings are not mere bodies: they are rational and autonomous beings, with (if the Christian teaching on this matter is correct) an essential orientation towards friendship with God in a life after this one. On this view, a health professional

---

[1]   This line of argument is defended, for example, by E. L. Bandman and B. Bandman in their *Nursing Ethics in the Life Span* (Norwalk, U.S.A., 1985), pp. 134–136. My comments in the next couple of pages amount to an argument against the view held by the Bandmans and others.

who failed to take account of his patient's whole nature as a person with an eternal destiny would be adopting a short-sighted and indeed distorted picture of man. Since a professional should serve the *whole* man, man as he actually is and not in some unreal state of abstraction, there can be nothing unprofessional about taking this special character of man and his destiny into account. But more generally, to communicate the truth (the moral truth, in this case) is to show authentic respect for another person – since the other can flourish only in so far as he lives according to the truth. Hence the Christian nurse cannot be expected to put her Christian faith to one side as soon as she comes on duty, on the pretext that this is "the professional thing to do". On the contrary, she would act unprofessionally in leaving her Christian faith out of account and dealing with her patients as if that faith were not true. There can, then, be no objection to the nurse's attempting to guide a patient along morally right lines. The fact that the decision about what is to be done is finally up to the patient cannot alter this truth. And the fact that the nurse must proceed in a reasonable and tactful way if she decides to offer moral guidance should not deter her from making such an attempt.

Issues in genetic counselling

Questions concerning the morality of abortion are at the heart of many of the moral difficulties arising in genetic counselling, especially those involving prenatal diagnosis. These difficulties arise largely because, while some genetically-caused deformities can, at present, be detected only after birth, there are some others which can be detected at a fairly early stage in pregnancy. Among the latter are certain conditions, such as Tay-Sachs disease, sickle-cell anaemia, thalassaemia and Huntington's chorea which involve very severe mental and physical retardation, gross impairment of bodily functioning and (except for Huntington's chorea, which first shows itself in adulthood) death within the early years of life. Other conditions such as Down's syndrome and retinoblastoma, which are not so catastrophic in their effects, can also be detected. Since these genetic conditions often result in a leakage of foetal cells into the amniotic fluid, amniocentesis can be used to detect them. Some other, non-genetic conditions such as spina bifida can be detected by raised levels of alpha-foeto-protein in the mother's bloodstream. If a genetic or non-genetic deformity is detected, the woman carrying the child can opt for abortion. Would she act rightly in doing so? One can readily understand a couple's aversion to the idea of having to spend many years, perhaps, caring for a severely disabled child, but the crucial moral question remains: Given that the child is already in existence, already alive *in utero*, can it be right to destroy it? Clearly the answer is No. The presence of severe disability is no more a justification for killing an unborn child than it is for killing one who is already born. Would it, then, be right for a nurse to assist in such procedures as amniocentesis, knowing that frequently the point of the exercise is to detect a genetic abnormality so that an abortion can take place? (An additional problem is that amniocentesis is not an absolutely safe procedure for the foetus, since in a small number of cases (between 0.5 and 1.5 per cent) it results in a miscarriage.) Since there appears to be very little possibility of amniocentesis being undertaken for genuinely therapeutic reasons in early pregnancy, so that practically all such procedures carried out then will be performed with abortion in view,[1] can a nurse conscientiously participate in this sort of work?

Admittedly, not all the procedures which take place in genetic counselling are carried out with abortion in mind. Part of the genetic counsellor's work, for instance, is that of counselling prospective parents who are carriers of certain conditions, or who have already had a handicapped child, about the advisability of having further children. Nor is abortion always in prospect in pre-natal diagnosis. A condition such as phenylketonuria, if diagnosed by means of an enzyme test while the infant is still *in utero*, can be treated by dietary means with complete success. Likewise, diagnosis of retinoblastoma in a child *in utero* will enable his parents to make early arrangements for surgery to take place after his birth. However, much genetic counselling work does involve acceptance of abortion as a legitimate option, and given the present easy availability and widespread acceptance of abortion, the attitude expressible as "If I find that the unborn child has Down's syndrome [or Tay-Sachs disease, or thalassaemia, etc.], I can then have it aborted" is common also among patients. Indeed, many counselling clinics advise that those pregnant women who would not be prepared to countenance abortion should not apply for genetic counselling at all.[2] So although in principle genetic

---

1. See, e.g., Sr. Regis Mary Dunne, "Genetic Counselling", in J. N. Santamaria (ed.), *Life in Our Power* (Melbourne, 1983), pp. 35–44, at p. 42.

2. For example, a circular issued to patients at a London hospital on "Screening for Spina Bifida" gives brief details of the various tests offered, and then states: "If as a result of these investigations it seems probable that there is a neural tube defect, you will be offered a termination of pregnancy. If you and your husband would not contemplate termination of pregnancy, then we suggest that you do not embark upon these tests at all."

counselling has many morally proper uses, in practice abortion is so widely accepted these days that a nurse who recognizes the evil of abortion would be foolish and wrong to take up this line of work. Only if she were able to work for a clinic whose staff were committed to oppose abortion would all ground of objection be removed.[1]

Care for the handicapped new-born

In 1975, Dr. John Lorber, of the Department of Paediatrics at the University of Sheffield, published an article, "Ethical Problems in the Management of Myelomeningocele and Hydrocephalus", which has been widely read and commented upon. Dr. Lorber's argument focused on new-born babies suffering from very severe cases of myelomeningocele (the commonest form of spina bifida, in which the spinal cord protrudes through the cystic sac), which usually give rise to hydrocephalus. These neonates, he argued, have such a low quality of life that they should have all forms of life-prolonging treatment withdrawn from them. They should be kept warm and comfortable and "fed on demand"; but apart from this, nothing should be done to prolong their lives.[2] The ideas of Dr. (later Professor) Lorber were implemented at his own paediatric unit in Sheffield, and many other such units probably operate along similar lines today. Writing some years after his original article, Dr. Lorber defended his proposals in the following way:

> ... once parents of a severely affected child know what kind of life their baby faces and what its handicaps will almost certainly be, almost 100 per cent are against treatment, and would be even if the doctor were to try to persuade them to agree to an operation and other treatment...
>
> The survival of extremely affected individuals has a major effect on family life. Mental breakdown in the parents is not rare, and sometimes leads to suicide. The divorce rate and family break-up is much higher than in the general population. The brothers and sisters of the

---

[1.] Ethical problems raised by ante-natal screening are examined in detail in Agneta Sutton's book *Ethical Problems in Pre-Natal Diagnosis*, to be published by the Linacre Centre in 1989.

[2.] J. Lorber, "Ethical Problems in the Management of Myelomeningocele and Hydrocephalus", *Journal of the Royal College of Physicians*, vol. 10, no. 1, 1975, pp. 47–60.

handicapped child suffer and there are major financial implications for a family, even when treatment is free.[1]

In practice, what has happened in many hospitals is that when parents and paediatrician have agreed that a baby should not be treated, the baby has been denied all feeding apart from water, and has been sedated with a drug such as chloral hydrate so that he will not suffer from pangs of hunger. Hence his death, which will occur within a fortnight or there-abouts, will most likely be from starvation. Someone attempting to justify this treatment of a defective neonate might argue as follows. "The parents should consider the severity of the child's condition and try to assess the quality of life it will have if it is treated and enabled to live for a certain (more or less long) period. Would it suffer greatly from pain and discomfort? Would its ability to move around be severely limited? Would it be denied all sorts of everyday pleasures which most children can take for granted? If the answer to all these questions is Yes, the conclusion must be that the new-born child could never have an adequate quality of life, and hence should not be encouraged to live. To this end, not only should he be denied any aggressive medical treatment − medicines, operations, artificial life support − but he should not even be fed. He should be kept warm and comfortable, with the help of sedatives, until he eventually dies of starvation."

This regime, sometimes called "nursing care only", was the one followed by Dr. Leonard Arthur in a case which led to a court action in 1981. Dr. Arthur had recommended that a baby with Downs syndrome, born at Derby City Hospital in June, 1980, should be given "nursing care only". The child, named John Pearson, was kept continuously sedated and given water only until he eventually died at the age of three days. Nutrition was withheld from him precisely because it would have kept him alive. The Director of Public Prosecutions subsequently took legal action against Dr. Arthur, charging him with attempted murder of the child. Dr. Arthur was, however, acquitted in November, 1981.[2] It is important to note that baby John Pearson was not afflicted by duodenal atresia, as sometimes happens to Down's syndrome babies, and there was therefore no natural obstacle to feeding him in the normal way. The

---

[1]   J. Lorber, "Commentary 1 and Reply", *Journal of Medical Ethics*, vol. 7, 1981, p. 121.

[2]   See the account of this case in "Note: Regina v. Arthur", an appendix to the report of the Linacre Centre's Working Party, *Euthanasia and Clinical Practice*, pp. 85–88.

parents' intention in refusing any "active treatment" of him was clearly *that he should die*; and it is arguable that the same intention must have motivated Dr. Arthur himself and the nurses who cared for the baby during his three days of life.

Paediatric nurses play a crucial role in cases such as this, because although it is the consultant paediatrician who decides that a new-born child should be given this minimal treatment, it is the nursing staff who have to put his decision into effect. It is they who have to be near to the baby all the time that they are on duty, while he is slowly dying through starvation. (It is reported that baby John Pearson received only one visit from a doctor after Dr. Arthur had directed that he be given "nursing care only". This visit "was from a senior house officer who asked to be told when the child died so that specimens could be taken from him."[1]) Since nurses are supposed to carry out the paediatrician's order, they must decide whether what they are being asked to do is or is not morally acceptable.

What makes this problem often especially difficult is that much depends upon the extent to which a handicapped new-born baby will actually be benefited by any proposed medical treatment, and that this is, to some extent at least, a matter on which one must rely on the paediatrician's judgment. He is the expert on the conditions from which babies can suffer, and the type of treatment (if any) which is effective in countering those conditions. Normally, then, when he expresses a judgment on some purely medical matter – on (say) the nature and severity of the condition of this particular new-born child, or on the effectiveness of various ways of treating that condition – the layman and the paediatric nurse will accept what he has to say. The situation changes, however, when the paediatrician expresses some opinion about the overall "worthwhileness", or lack of it, of the life of a child after receiving treatment, or on the moral justification or otherwise of sustaining his life. Here the paediatrician is speaking outside the narrow area in which he has professional competence, and his point of view may be no more expert or informed or well-balanced than that of the average man in the street. He may, in fact, be every bit as prone to act out of sheer prejudice as anybody else. This point is important because some paediatricians, like many people in society at large, hold views on the question of what constitutes a worthwhile life which are, to say the least, disputable.

[1.] *Euthanasia and Clinical Practice*, p. 85.

Relying upon the moral principles outlined in earlier chapters, what can we say about the duties of doctors and nurses to treat handicapped new-born children? The most important principle here is that any action or omission which is aimed at bringing about the death of an innocent human being is wrong. This general principle is as readily applicable to the treatment of handicapped babies as to that of adults; and it rules out decisively the practice of denying all nourishment to severely handicapped infants and sedating them so that they will die as quickly as possible. Since the motive for withdrawing all life-prolonging measures is precisely that the babies should die, we have here a death-dealing intention; and this death-dealing intention is sufficient to make the treatment amount to homicide. It would be sheer confusion to think that the fact that one is not actively intervening to kill these infants – by giving them a lethal injection, say – but is simply "standing back and letting them die" means that one is acting rightly. For, as we saw in Chapter Seven, *the intention that somebody die* is sufficient to make a given line of conduct homicidal, regardless of whether the victim's death is brought about by active intervention or by omission. So the resort to "nursing care only" in the treatment of severely handicapped babies is untenable; on this point we can agree with those hard-headed advocates of killing by positive action, such as John Harris,[1] Peter Singer and Helga Kuhse[2] that when one has decided to bring about a patient's death, any supposed moral superiority of non-treatment over active intervention is illusory. If, moreover, we deal with problems of this sort on the basis of the distinction between ordinary and extraordinary means of treatment, we see that there can be no justification at all for "nursing care only"; for here the provision of nutrition could hardly be regarded as an extraordinary means of treatment: it does not create any great burden for the child or anyone else, and it benefits him at least to the extent of enabling him to live a little longer – perhaps considerably longer – than would otherwise have been possible.

Evidentally, then, the principle that it is wrong to kill intentionally an innocent person rules out the treatment of Down's syndrome baby John Pearson by Dr. Leonard Arthur and those of his medical and nursing colleagues who were directly involved in the "care" of the child. For these

---

[1] J. Harris, "Ethical problems in the management of some severely handicapped children", *Journal of Medical Ethics*, vol. 7, no. 3, 1981, pp. 117–120.
[2] H. Kuhse and P. Singer, *Should the Baby Live?* (Oxford, 1985).

health professionals acted as they did in order to bring it about that baby John Pearson would die. It is this intention that death be brought about which renders unacceptable the action of Dr. Arthur and his colleagues. By contrast, omission of treatment reasonably judged to be ethically extraordinary would not fall victim to this objection.

Consider now a situation in which a Down's syndrome baby is suffering from duodenal atresia, that is, a blockage of the duodenum which prevents him from digesting food. The operation to remove such a blockage is a standard procedure, and in the case of a baby born with duodenal atresia but with no other handicap, the surgical team would remove it without hesitation. If, then, the parents of a Down's syndrome baby decide against having the atresia rectified and their paediatric surgeon concurs with this decision, this can only be because they want the baby to die precisely because it is a Down's syndrome baby. Here we have a refusal of treatment which is motivated by a death-dealing intention and is therefore morally wrong. The situation would admittedly be different for a child suffering from Down's syndrome and duodenal atresia together with various other handicaps from which he would inevitably die within a short time; it might then reasonably be decided that subjecting him to surgery would impose too great a burden by comparison with the small benefit which the surgery would make available to him, and this decision would be innocent of any death-dealing intent. But in the absence of these additional conditions, surgery to rectify the atresia would evidently be an ordinary means, for it would greatly benefit the baby – by enabling him to live for many years rather than a few days – and would normally impose no unduly severe burden on him or on anyone else.

In general, when the treatment of a handicapped baby is at issue, the crucial question is: Are this baby's physical and/or mental abilities so severely impaired that the surgical or other procedures which might be proposed for treating them are extraordinary means – either because they promise only minimal benefit, or because the treatment itself would involve serious hardship to the child which would not be justified by any foreseeable benefit to him? If the answer is Yes, parents can rightly request that such treatment not be given, and paediatricians and nurses will act rightly in acting in accord with such requests. But if something can be done to help a handicapped baby without imposing any great burden on him, parents are obliged to request that that treatment be given; a paediatrician would act wrongly in withholding the treatment, with or without the consent of the parents. Nurses would be obliged not to provide "nursing care only" for the baby, for if they did do this they would be sharing the paediatrician's immoral death-dealing intention.

Even for an experienced paediatric nurse it may, however, be difficult to determine whether a child's condition is really such that a proposed surgical or other treatment would be ethically extraordinary. Provided that there are no definite grounds for doubting the paediatrician's *medical* judgment about the benefits and harms of the proposed treatment, and providing that his proposals are based on that medical judgment rather than on other, more disputable, grounds, a nurse would act rightly in co-operating with his decision. She would have reason not to co-operate only if the paediatrician's judgment seemed manifestly unreasonable or if she suspected that he was deciding the fate of an infant on the basis of a mistaken belief about what makes for an acceptable quality of life – for example, that life is not worth living if one is suffering from Down's syndrome. It should be added here that it may not be easy to determine whether someone's decisions and actions are based on wrong-headed beliefs of this sort. Certainly this is the case if someone says quite generally that life for a Down's syndrome or spina bifida child is not of sufficiently high quality to justify one in keeping it going. But if a paediatrician says of an individual patient, "This child could never have a worthwhile life", or even "This child would be better off dead", he may or may not be giving vent to wrong attitudes towards those suffering from grave handicaps. Such statements are, to say the least, offensive; but it is possible that in saying (e.g.) "This child would be better off dead" a doctor might mean no more than: "Nothing we could do for this child would really benefit him, so it is better to let him die". It would, then, be wrong to place too much emphasis on comments such as these. They may express an immoral attitude to new-born life, but then again they may not. This is certainly an area in which a refusal to jump to conclusions, as well as a willingness to talk matters over with one's nursing colleagues – and also with the paediatrician, if this is a practical option – are valuable aids to a nurse in attempting to decide on the right course of action.

★   ★   ★

This Chapter in Summary

The subject of abortion raises some serious problems of co-operation for nurses. In examining the morality or otherwise of abortion, one has to answer the question: "Is the human foetus a human being, a person in the full sense of the word?" If we answer Yes, we are also committed to saying that abortion is one of those acts which are morally wrong in principle, wrong "whatever the consequences". It is argued here that the foetus is a person in the full sense, one which differs from those beings which more obviously count as persons only in being a radically immature member of the human race. The widespread idea that the foetus is only a potential person arises from a confusion of the notion of immaturity with that of potentiality. It follows that abortion is an intrinsically wrong act, and hence that there are severe limits to the material co-operation of nurses in abortion procedures. (Formal co-operation is, of course, always wrong.) The fact that genetic counselling tends nowadays to presuppose the abortion of handicapped foetuses as a morally legitimate option makes it unlikely that the nurse who opposes abortion could commit herself to this work. Concerning the treatment of handicapped new-born children, we have to say that any attempt to bring about the death of these children, whether through deliberate killing or omission of life-preserving treatment, is morally wrong. A difficulty here, however, is that it is sometimes not easy to decide from the remarks of (say) a consultant paediatrician whether a baby's death is in fact being aimed at in a particular case. It would be unwise to jump to conclusions on matters such as this, although careful reflexion should reveal what is at stake in most cases.

CHAPTER THIRTEEN

ISSUES IN SEXUAL ETHICS

At first sight, problems of sexual morality might appear not to affect the nurse's work to any great extent. For these problems belong to an essentially private area of people's lives, in which what is at stake is usually an intimate relationship between two individual persons. But it is evident that many of the ethical problems already discussed – problems of confidentiality, for instance – will arise with special urgency in an area such as sexuality which has to do with people's most private thoughts and actions. And in recent times, especially since the development and wide-spread use of new methods of birth prevention, doctors and nurses have found themselves facing a number of contentious moral issues. The so-called contraceptive pill is the best-known of these new methods of birth prevention, but other devices and techniques – intra-uterine devices, for example – have also come to be widely used. In addition, sterilization, both male and female, is now a common procedure in hospitals. Moral problems are raised not only by attempts to prevent childbirth but also by certain means of achieving pregnancy, particularly artificial insemination and *in vitro* fertilization. To deal satisfactorily with these problems, we have to answer such questions as: What is the sort of context in which it is appropriate for human sexual activity to take place? Is the relationship of marriage especially important in this regard?; and: What relation should hold between sexual intercourse and the procreation of new life?

Four distinct areas of nursing work which inevitably pose questions of sexual morality are those concerning contraception, sterilization, artificial insemination and *in vitro* fertilization. The Catholic nurse is bound to realize the acuteness of these problems, because the Church's teachings on sexual ethics make co-operation in these practices morally dubious, to say the least. Two such Catholic teachings are especially important: first, that sexual activity needs to be placed squarely in the context of marriage and family life, and secondly, that sexual intercourse and procreation must be seen as inseparably bound up with each other, so that it would be wrong to attempt to separate them in practice. Both these teachings run contrary to the permissive attitude towards sexuality which is currently wide-spread, so a Catholic nurse who upholds the Church's teachings may encounter serious problems of co-operation if she is assigned tasks connected with contraception, say, or sterilization.

The two "meanings" of sexual activity

If the practices mainly under consideration here – contraception, sterilization, artificial insemination and *in vitro* fertilization – were morally good or at least neutral, no nurse would ever experience difficulties of co-operation in their regard. It is because, on the Catholic view, all four practices are objectionable that such problems are inescapable. We need, then, to look more closely at the grounds for the Church's attitude towards these practices; and this means that we must first look at the general Catholic attitude to human sexuality, since it is this which grounds the conclusions defended by Catholic moralists about the morality or immorality of particular practices. Consider the following passage, from the most recent magisterial document on sexual ethics, the instruction *Donum Vitae*, issued in March, 1987:

> The Church's teaching on marriage and human procreation affirms the "inseparable connection, willed by God and unable to be broken by man on his own initiative, between the two meanings of the conjugal act: the unitive meaning and the procreative meaning. Indeed, by its intimate structure, the conjugal act, while most closely uniting husband and wife, capacitates them for the generation of new lives, according to laws inscribed in the very being of man and of woman.". . .

> The same doctrine concerning the link between the meanings of the conjugal act and between the goods of marriage throws light on the moral problem of. . . [artificial insemination and *in vitro* fertilization], since "it is never permitted to separate these different aspects to such a degree as positively to exclude either the procreative intention or the conjugal relation."[1]

---

[1]. Sacred Congregation for the Doctrine of the Faith (S.C.D.F.), *Instruction of Respect for Human Life in its Origin and on the Dignity of Procreation* (*Donum Vitae*) (Vatican City, 1987), pp. 26–27. The first internal quotation is from Pope Paul VI's encyclical *Humanae Vitae* (1968), and the second is from a discourse given by Pope Pius XII in 1956.

The key assertion here is that the sexual intercourse of a married couple (or "the conjugal act", as the document terms it) is an act with two distinct but closely-associated intelligible aspects or "meanings", a unitive meaning and a procreative meaning. On this view, sexual activity should be seen not as just a piece of physical behaviour, a mere coupling of bodies, but in relation to the whole nature of man, spiritual as well as physical. On the one hand, the sexual act is *unitive*, that is, it expresses the love and mutual commitment of the spouses, their shared life together and their commitment to each other for the future. On the other hand the sexual act is *procreative*, that is, it carries an essential reference to the procreation of new life, because the love between the partners which it expresses is not centred solely upon themselves, but is open to the possibility of the "gift" of a child who will enter into their lives as, in a sense, the embodiment of that mutual love and commitment.

This assertion of the procreative character of sexual activity is rejected by many people today. They will quite happily admit the unitive character of sexual intercourse, since they realize that sexual intercourse which expresses no abiding love or commitment between the partners but consists merely in procuring sexual pleasure is a distorted form of sexual activity, promising no lasting fulfilment or happiness to either partner. But they may reject in the following way the idea that sexual activity has an intrinsically procreative "meaning" or "significance": "Admittedly, in the normal course of events sexual intercourse is the way we bring other human beings into existence, but this procreative effect is possible only for a few days during a woman's menstrual cycle, and so the great majority of sexual acts do not lead to the conception of a child. Why, then, assert that the conjugal act *always* has this 'procreative meaning'? And surely this talk of 'procreative meaning' amounts to no more than this: that as a matter of fact, sexual intercourse, if engaged in at certain times, is capable of bringing it about that a child is conceived. But if this is all that it means, isn't the phrase 'procreative meaning' an unnecessarily pretentious way of referring to it?"

Objections along these lines are not easy to rebut, because the conclusion that sexual activity has these two "meanings", the unitive and the procreative, is not drawn directly from premises founded on biological data, but is rather the expression of what we might call a whole way of looking at things. An advocate of the Catholic position might reply as follows: "I can't *prove* from neutral premises, so to speak, that the good which is at stake in sexual activity is that common life of mutual commitment which essentially involves openness to the gift of new life and is to be found fully present only in the context of life-long marriage. In the same way, I can't prove that knowledge and health and friendship are basic human goods. I do claim, however, that if one conducts one's sexual life with respect for what the Church calls the two fundamental 'meanings' of the sexual act, one will naturally come to see that these two 'meanings' are appropriately regarded as the Catholic tradition regards them. The kind of knowledge which one will then have of the significance of human sexual life will differ from the purely 'exterior', objective knowledge which we acquire when we use our sensory organs. It will rather be an instance of what Christian philosophers have often called, following St. Thomas Aquinas, connatural knowledge – that is, a type of knowledge which is had 'from the inside' and which follows upon the fact that we are living the sort of life which is appropriate for a being of human nature.[1] It will then be clear that human sexual activity has to do both with expressing mutual love and commitment and with openness to the procreation of new life, and that the alternative view, which cuts off the sexual act from any intrinsic connexion with procreation, is an impoverished conception of what that act is all about, something which views a part of human sexuality as if it were the whole." One could go on to suggest that the admitted difficulty of recognizing the essentially procreative character of sexual activity is hardly surprising if one views the matter in the light of Christian teaching about man's fallen state. For a consequence of original sin is concupiscence, that unruliness of man's sensual impulses which can cloud his understanding and impede the operation of his reason; and as a result, man's sexual impulses are all too easily accepted as having no significance beyond the provision of immediate pleasure to their possessor. In fact, a promiscuous man or woman would probably want to carry further the line of argument against the Catholic position which was formulated earlier. That argument, while not granting the sexual act any procreative significance, did

---

[1.] For a brief account of what this "connatural knowledge" amounts to, see J. Maritain, *The Range of Reason* (London, 1953), Chapter Three, "On Knowledge through Connaturality" (pp. 22–29). Maritain says (p. 23) that "In this knowledge through union or inclination, connaturality or congeniality, the intellect is at play not alone, but together with affective inclinations and the dispositions of the will, and is guided and directed by them. It is not rational knowledge, knowledge through the conceptual, logical and discursive exercise of reason. But it is really and genuinely knowledge, though obscure and perhaps incapable of giving account of itself, or of being translated into words."

concede to it a unitive significance; the promiscuous person, however, will refuse to admit even this much. He will say that although sexual activity *can* express the love and mutual commitment of man and woman, it does not have to do so, but can legitimately be a vehicle for bringing sexual pleasure to any couple who wish to strike up a temporary liaison. The point here is that the essentially unitive character of sexual intercourse can no more be established by arguing from "neutral" premises than can the essentially procreative character or meaning of the sexual act. To say this is not to rule out any possibility of reaching the truth about these controverted issues; it is, rather, to indicate that the truth of the matter may have to be simply "seen" or apprehended connaturally, by those whose way of life and thought is already properly integrated, or on the way to being integrated, by respect for the basic goods of human life. And since, on the Christian view, this connatural apprehension is by no means easy to obtain, given the disruption caused by concupiscence to our ability to think clear-headedly about these things, it is appropriate that the Church should attempt to guide us about the nature of the human goods which are really at stake in sexual activity.

There also appear to be some sound *negative* arguments for the conclusion that human sexual activity has a procreative as well as a unitive meaning. Suppose, for example, that the objector is correct and that sexual intercourse has no intrinsic procreative meaning or significance at all. In that case, why should it be supposed that sexual partners should have to be *exclusive* and *lifelong* sexual partners, committed to each other by the promises made in contracting marriage? Why should a man or woman not feel free to enter a number of temporary liaisons, or to conduct several extra-marital affairs simultaneously? There seem to be no grounds for ruling out these things. Likewise, why not accept homosexual relations, or sexual activity with children, provided that in all such cases the partners consent? If, on the other hand, sexual intercourse is intrinsically bound up with procreation, and if, also, the begetting and raising of children is appropriate only in the context of a single man-woman couple who undertake an unshakable commitment to care for their children, we can see *why* extra-marital affairs, homosexual practices and pederasty are to be condemned. So unless someone is prepared to argue that such practices are, in fact, all morally proper, he will have to admit that the connexion between sexual activity and procreation is much closer than he was at first prepared to admit; and this amounts to saying that there is indeed a procreative meaning or significance to sexual intercourse, in addition to its unitive meaning.

Let us now inquire what sort of moral appraisal should be given of the four practices which primarily interest us: contraception, sterilization, artificial insemination and *in vitro* fertilization.

Contraception

A couple who use contraceptives to render their sexual act infertile are, in effect, acting to deprive the sexual act of one of its essential aspects, its procreative meaning or significance; and this destruction of procreative significance has traditionally been regarded as morally wrong in the Catholic moral tradition. By contrast, a couple who, for sound reasons, do not wish to have a child at a given stage in their lives, and therefore confine their sexual activity to those days when a child cannot be conceived, are not deliberately depriving the sexual act of something essentially belonging to it. They are not, then, setting their will against the integral sexual act, understood as comprising procreative as well as unitive significance, and hence their action is in no way morally objectionable.

These comments make it clear that the traditional condemnation of all attempts to destroy the procreative character or meaning of freely-chosen sexual intercourse is claimed to be founded on the nature of things, the way things are. What people often carelessly refer to as "the Catholic Church's ban on contraception" is in fact a Catholic *teaching* that freely-chosen sexual intercourse which is deliberately rendered sterile is an intrinsically wrong act and would be so even if the Church had never made any official pronouncement on the subject.

Note that what is evil, on this view, is not the taking of contraceptive measures as such, but the taking of such measures to render infertile an act of sexual intercourse which is freely engaged in. The teaching is that it is wrong to engage deliberately in the sexual act and at the same time to deprive that act of its procreative meaning. But a woman who has been raped, for instance, has not made a choice which is simultaneously for sexual activity but against procreation. Hence, if she takes contraceptive measures to avoid pregnancy as a result of having been raped, she is not setting her will against the integral sexual good at all: she is rather, and quite legitimately, attempting to counter the continuing effects of the assault on her and the unjust invasion of her body. So when people say "The Catholic Church teaches that contraception is morally evil and not to be engaged in" they are, in fact, oversimplifying. More accurately, the Church condemns, not contraception *tout court*, but rather contracepted sexual intercourse which is freely chosen, or, to express it as clearly as possible, sexual intercourse in which a person engages freely, but which he or she deliberately attempts to render infertile.

It is important to distinguish between the Catholic Church's teaching about contraception, and, on the other hand, the arguments which individual theologians and philosophers may expound in support of that teaching. It has recently been argued that the consistency of this teaching over the years, and its acceptance by Catholic bishops throughout the world, is sufficient to make it an infallible teaching of the Church's ordinary magisterium.[1] Moreover, the rejection of contraceptive intercourse made by Paul VI in *Humanae Vitae* has on many occasions been strongly defended and restated by John Paul II. As far as the Catholic Church is concerned, then, the condemnation of contraception is evidently here to stay; and it is arguable that a Catholic who really believes that the Church's is able to pronounce decisively on contentious doctrinal and moral issues will be impelled to accept the Church's consistent teaching simply because that is what it is. However, an exclusive reliance on the Church's authority is clearly a less-than-perfect option, for if contracepted intercourse is indeed wrong, it is not wrong because the Church says so but because of what it is in itself. And in this case it should be possible for us to catch some glimpse, at least, of the reason why it is wrong.[2] The Church's *magisterium*, when it is reiterating a teaching which

---

1. Cf. J. C. Ford, S.J., and G. G. Grisez, "Contraception and the Infallibility of the Ordinary Magisterium", in *Theological Studies*, vol. 39, 1978, pp. 263–267, and also J. M. Finnis, "Infallibility", in J. N. Santamaria and J. J. Billings (eds.), *Human Love and Human Life* (Melbourne, 1979), pp. 167–183. Finnis says (p. 171): "Even if the teaching proposed in *Humanae Vitae* is not infallibly defined in that document, that same teaching may be an infallible teaching of the Church. Indeed, I think it certainly is." The Catholic teaching concerning the infallibility of the ordinary magisterium is set out in paragraph 25 of the Second Vatican Council's apostolic constitution *Lumen Gentium*: "Although the bishops individually do not enjoy the prerogative of infallibility, they nevertheless proclaim the teaching of Christ infallibly, even when they are dispersed throughout the world, provided that they remain in communion with each other and with the successor of Peter and that in authoritatively teaching on matters of faith and morals they agree in one judgment as to that to be held definitively."

2. Cf. The following remarks of Dietrich von Hildebrand in his *The Encyclical Humanae Vitae: A Sign of Contradiction* (Chicago, 1969), p. xiii: "It is. . . important that [faithful married Catholics] understand the true *reason* for the sinfulness of artificial birth control; for the more clearly a person perceives why a thing is sinful, the more easily he will be able to avoid the sin even at the price of great sacrifice – although the Church's unequivocal prohibition should alone

has been taught consistently over the years, is often content to restate the teaching itself with such precisions and new emphases as are required, rather than with producing an argument which might convince a sceptic. Sometimes, also, theologians differ among themselves about the best way of defending a given point of Church teaching, and in this case the Church itself may be concerned to leave this secondary question – "How is the teaching to be defended?" – open. This is, in fact, what Paul VI appears to have done in *Humanae Vitae*.[1] At any rate, we need to ask whether there are grounds for accepting the Church's condemnation of contracepted intercourse, grounds which can be appreciated by someone who is not a Catholic and who is therefore not inclined to accept the teaching on contraception simply on the Church's authority.

Here we come up against a real difficulty. For it is undeniable that what lies behind the recent widespread rejection of the Church's teaching, and not only by non-Catholics, is that these people simply do not see anything wrong with what the Church condemns. So we have the sort of situation to which media commentators drew our attention during Pope John Paul II's visit to the U.S.A. in 1987: that a large proportion of Americans who claim to be Catholics believe that contracepted intercourse within marriage is perfectly acceptable. It may well be, of course, that these people have been so badly affected by the pressures and prevailing attitudes of a technologically-orientated and materialistic society that they can no longer "see" something which should be obvious to them. But if, as the Church maintains, the evil of contracepted intercourse is an objective fact about that very human act itself, it should be possible for ordinary people, even in this day and age, to apprehend that this is so. Can we advance any argument which might help them to do this?

One line of argument which has recently been defended relies on the principle that it is wrong directly to attack one of the basic human goods. For (the argument runs) life-in-its-transmission is either itself a basic good or an integral "part" of some basic good – since the procreation of

suffice for the faithful, since obedience to a divine command does not depend on one's understanding the reason for it."

[1] See J. M. Finnis, "Natural Law and Unnatural Acts", in *The Heythrop Journal*, vol. XI, no. 4, October, 1970, pp. 365–387, at p. 386: "The encyclical [*sc.*, *Humanae Vitae*] suffers, I think, from three general weaknesses of presentation. The first is its evident desire to avoid saying anything that would close the debate between three main schools of thought about the proper way of explaining the Christian doctrine on anti-procreative choices. . ."

new life is clearly one of those activities which are good in themselves, good intrinsically rather than good as means to something else – and contracepted intercourse consists in one's setting oneself deliberately against this good. Just as it is wrong to murder someone because in doing this one deliberately sets out to deprive one's victim of a basic human good, the good of life, so it is wrong to use contraceptives to prevent conception because one thereby sets oneself against the good of life-in-its-transmission. One of the most thorough recent surveys of this whole area, the volume *Catholic Sexual Ethics* by Lawler, Boyle and May, expresses the argument as follows:

> In contraceptive intercourse one chooses both to have sexual intercourse and to prevent the act from being procreative. The contraceptive element in the dual act is aimed precisely and directly against the possible coming-to-be of human life. As the American bishops note [in their pastoral letter *To Live in Christ Jesus*], such a prevention is a rejection of the "life-giving meaning of intercourse"; and "the wrongness of such an act lies in the rejection of this value."

> Three major steps can be noted in the argument to establish this point. First, the procreative good is intrinsically and always good. Second, a contraceptive deed acts directly against this good, and of itself does nothing but assail that good. Third, it is always immoral to so act directly against a basic human good.[1]

Later on, the authors draw the following comparisons between contracepted intercourse and other wrong acts:

> ... The logic and pattern of contraceptive acts is like that of perjury committed for "good reasons". In such perjury one attacks truth in an act (an oath) which of its very nature is ordered to the truth, perhaps on the grounds that by doing so one might prevent a "dangerous truth" from doing harm. This is not like seeking to avoid the harm by remaining silent, for in the latter case one honours the truth by refusing to attack it. Again, contraception is like euthanasia (mercy killing) in its logical structure. In mercy killing one chooses to kill, to act directly against innocent life, for

---

1. R. Lawler, J. Boyle and W. E. May, *Catholic Sexual Ethics* (Huntington, U.S.A., 1985), p. 159.

the sake of removing the burdens of a painful or debilitated existence. One chooses against life for the sake of what seem to be noble purposes.

In a contraceptive act, one freely and deliberately chooses to attack a great human good. The motive for this act may be upright; one may wish to avoid for oneself and others the harms that would be inseparable from the untimely realization of that good. But there are many ways in which those harms could be avoided, some good and some evil.[1]

Is this argument sound? It could be urged that it fails to show contracepted intercourse to be intrinsically wrong. Consider again a situation considered in Chapter Six. A mother stops her child from playing in the garden and brings her inside so that she will eat her lunch. Does the mother act wrongly by directly attacking the basic good of play in the person of her child? Surely not: she could be said to attack this good directly only if she were systematically to deprive the child of opportunities to play, either with friends or by herself, on an unreasonably high number of occasions. To stop her from playing on a single occasion, or even regularly – if, for example, the child tends to want to play when she should be doing other things – is not necessarily to do her any wrong. Similarly, it could be argued, a couple who use contraceptives in order to prevent procreation do not act directly against the good of life-in-its-transmission, provided they have adequate grounds for doing so; that is, that their desire to avoid conceiving a child at this particular time is reasonable. Whether or not a couple act against the good of life-in-its-transmission is, on this view, to be ascertained by determining, not whether they act to prevent conception from taking place on any one occasion, but whether or not they have shown themselves to be insufficiently open to this great good *over the whole course of their married life*. As one critic of the Catholic position has expressed it:

> One of the arguments in favour of artificial contraception which Paul VI's famous encyclical mentioned, but did not answer, was. . . that the sexual life of a married couple should be viewed as a whole, not in terms of its distinct acts of intercourse. . . To break marriage down into a series of disconnected sexual acts is to falsify its true

---

[1] *Catholic Sexual Ethics*, pp. 161–2.

nature. As a whole, then, the married love of any couple should (barring serious reasons to the contrary) be both relation-building and procreative. . . But it is artificial to insist, as *Humanae Vitae* did, that 'each and every marriage act' must express the two goods equally.[1]

What the response of Boyle, Lawler and May would be to this objection I do not know, but I cannot myself see that their position is capable of withstanding it. Instead of trying to patch up their argument it is better, I believe, to rely on a quite different approach. A key consideration here is the conception of the nature of man which is part of Catholic teaching but which is also supported by philosophical reasoning, since it is defensible on the basis of facts about man and his characteristic activities which are available to all men, whether they are Christians or not. This conception involves two essential theses: first, that man is a composite of matter and a spiritual soul; and secondly, that the soul is that which explains, not only the fact that man has the higher mental abilities of thinking, deliberating and willing, but also that his body *is* a human body with its appropriate physical characteristics and abilities. Given that the human soul is a *spiritual* soul – that is, that it is not composed of any sort of matter but belongs to an entirely different order – it cannot be produced by any physical process but must be created directly by God.[2] This means that procreation is not an activity which a couple carry out all by themselves, but involves an intimate co-operation with God Himself: there is, then, what we could call a specifically religious dimension of human procreation. In a sense, all human activity is activity in which God co-operates, because human beings could not exist or act at all if they were not continuously sustained in existence by God's creative power – and the same is true of all animal and plant and mineral activity. But procreation involves a very special kind of co-operation with God, because in procreation God uses the matter which is provided by the two parents, infusing into that matter a human soul which is a distinct spiritual being in its own right, and which He has created out of nothing specially for this occasion. So in procreation we have an activity which, because it involves

---

[1]   O. O'Donovan, *Begotten or Made?* (Oxford, 1984), pp. 76–7.

[2]   See Pope Pius XII's encyclical *Humani Generis* (1950). St. Thomas Aquinas defends this view of man's nature in the *Summa Theologiae*, part 1, questions 75–89, while Josef Pieper's *Death and Immortality* (London, 1969) is a valuable modern discussion of this traditional account of the nature and function of the human soul.

the creative activity of God in a way which goes far beyond His general conservation of creatures in being, is invested with a specially holy or sacred character. It is not a purely mundane transaction between man and woman but an act in which man and woman together co-operate with God. Admittedly, God's intervention does not take place until some time after the couple's sexual act, so it could be argued that their sexual activity does not have this sacred aspect until God creates and imparts the soul – at fertilization, let us say. But the fact that God *is going* to intervene in this way must surely change our estimation of the significance of human sexual activity as it is even before God joins matter and soul: given that this act of sexual intercourse will, if nature is allowed to take its course, be "crowned" by a special act of divine creation, it must be seen in a different light from any purely physical and man-dependent process: it is *already* a co-operative act in virtue of what may become of it. Because this is what human sexual activity actually is, certain kinds of action which would be appropriate in the case of a wholly physical process of production brought about by the two parents are in fact inappropriate and immoral. One such action would be that of stopping the process after it had started: if one does this, one treats a process which is an intimate co-operation with God's creative activity as if it were subject to one's own exclusive jurisdiction. The fact that God *is* specially involved in procreation means that one should adopt towards that process an attitude of reverence akin to that which one adopts towards God Himself.

On this view the traditional prohibition against contracepted sexual intercourse is seen to make sense. To engage freely in sexual intercourse while using contraceptives to ensure that one's sexual act does not result in the conception of a child is to treat procreation as if it were an act of production which the couple carry out entirely by themselves, and which they might choose to carry through or to terminate as they wish. This attitude is not appropriate once procreation is seen for what it is, an intimate co-operation between man, woman and God. This way of looking at human procreation naturally goes along with a view of the child as a gift of God. For since the parents do not produce their child themselves but co-operate with God, Who provides the human soul by which the child is a human being with all the physical and mental characteristics proper to a human being, they clearly receive their child from Him: the child is a gift from God to them. This being so, the parents should remain open to receiving this great gift and should never treat it in a way which implicitly denies that it is a gift.[1]

The same judgment has to be made about sterilization, which consists in deliberately rendering a man or woman permanently incapable of initiating this co-operative activity. If it is wrong to frustrate a given process of human procreation which is already under way, it is also wrong to bring it about deliberately that no such process will ever be able to get under way. In both cases we have human beings disregarding the true character of human procreation and treating it as if it were an act of production carried out entirely through their own resources.

Contraception and nursing practice

A nurse may be involved in giving contraceptive advice to patients or may be directed to assist in the fitting of certain devices aimed at preventing childbirth, such as the coil or intra-uterine device (IUD). Even if she is never engaged expressly in this kind of work, it is likely that patients will occasionally ask her advice about methods of birth control. How should she act in situations like these? Should she agree to participate in teaching about contraception or in fitting contraceptive devices? In replying to her patients' queries about birth control, should she give those patients the information they want in a factual, value-free way, or should she express her own moral outlook?

Here there enters a complicating factor, namely that there are good grounds for believing that some devices commonly called contraceptives have in fact an abortifacient effect. Certainly this appears to be the case with the IUD, which probably works by setting up a constant scraping action against the wall of the uterus which renders the endometrium inhospitable to the fertilised ovum, so that the latter cannot implant. In other words, although the IUD may have a spermicidal effect which is genuinely contraceptive, it also acts to prevent the four- or five-day-old embryo from implanting in the womb. It is also suspected that the so-called contraceptive pill sometimes functions as an abortifacient. For it is thought that although the pill does often work by preventing ovulation from taking place, it has also a "back-up" capacity to change the constitution of the endometrium so that any embryo which has managed to come

---

[1].   For a more complete development of these lines of argument, see Dietrich von Hildebrand's *The Encyclical Humanae Vitae: A Sign of Contradiction*, esp. Part II, pp. 29–49.

into being despite its "front-line" contraceptive effect is prevented from implanting. If this is so, nurses who co-operate in ostensibly contraceptive activity or contraceptive counselling will often, whether they realize it or not, be co-operating in abortion procedures. This danger is even more obviously present for participation in some more recent developments in the "contraceptive" field, such as the "morning after" pill. But even apart from this complicating factor concerning abortion, the wrongness of contracepted sexual intercourse clearly rules out both the taking of the pill by the individual and any formal co-operation on a nurse's part in a patient's taking of it; and the same judgment applies concerning other types of contraceptive device.

May a nurse give information to patients about contraceptive measures? This is one of many issues on which the principles of co-operation need to be applied, and (as we saw in Chapter Seven) they cannot be applied rigidly or mechanically but must take account of each particular situation. Given that the imparting of information concerning contraception is something normally expected of a nurse or health visitor by her hospital or local health authority, it is reasonable to say that she may respond to a patient's request by providing information about contraception, provided that she does simply provide information and does not in any way encourage the patient to have recourse to contraceptive measures or assist her in doing so. Indeed, she should make clear her disapproval of such measures whenever this appears to be possible and appropriate (e.g., when the patient is not determined to resort to contraceptive measures, and seems receptive to alternative suggestions). She would also act rightly in commending natural family planning to her patients, since NFP is free from the moral objections incurred by contraception, and in addition is not damaging to a woman's health, as contraception sometimes is.

Sterilization

Sterilization can be carried out on either a man or a woman, and the procedure can have either a therapeutic or a contraceptive aim. The procedure is therapeutic when it is aimed at protecting the patient's life or general health. So, for instance, a woman who has undergone a mastectomy may also have her ovaries removed, even though they are functioning healthily, because the ovaries produce oestrogen, which contributes to causing various tumours. Similarly, a surgeon may treat a man suffering from cancer of the prostate gland by removing not only the prostate gland itself, but also his testes, even though they may be perfectly healthy. Removing the prostate gland is usually not sufficient to eradicate the cancer, which is stimulated by androgens produced in the testes; if, therefore, the testes are removed, the disease is much less likely to progress unabated. In both these cases we have sterilization which is therapeutic because it is carried out not in order to render the subject infertile (although this is, of course, what happens) but in order to safeguard and preserve his life and health. Here a principle which moral theologians have called *the principle of totality* comes into play: one's sexual organs are not independent living substances but parts of an individual human being, and their functioning is subordinated to that of the whole. Hence, if the whole organism is seriously threatened, and the threat can be overcome only by destroying or suppressing the functioning of these organs, one may legitimately take such a step.

Contraceptive sterilization, by contrast, is carried out precisely in order to prevent conception from taking place. So, for example, a couple decide that their family is already as large as they would like it to be, so they resort to sterilization to ensure that there are no further additions. Or a woman is told that her uterus is in such a frail state that child-bearing would be dangerous for her, and she is advised to have a hysterectomy so that she can avoid this danger. In both these cases, the intention is that the patient's acts of sexual intercourse should be rendered infertile. Here we have, then, the same anti-procreative resolve as in contraception, and this means that the same moral judgment has to be made about contraceptive sterilization as about contraception. While a woman who is advised not to conceive another child because of an unhealthy uterus certainly deserves sympathetic assistance from health professionals, she should not seek to deal with her problem by doing something which – because it involves intentionally destroying an essential part of the significance of the sexual act – is in itself wrong. It can be concluded that any nurse who recognizes contraceptive sterilization as morally wrong will realize that she may not take part in sterilization procedures or co-operate formally in them.

Sterilization procedures are often carried out by a team consisting of a surgeon, an anaesthetist and two nurses, one assisting the surgeon and the other assisting the anaesthetist. Where this happens, both nurses evidently co-operate formally in the procedure. If, then, the operation is a contraceptive sterilization the nurses will both act wrongly. Material co-operation, on the other hand, would seem to encompass two kinds of acts: first, pre-medication, and secondly, some acts of giving information. It is at least arguable that pre-medication is so "close" to the procedure itself that it would, under almost all circumstances, be wrong to take part in it, unless the nursing care provided is a sort of "lowest-common-denominator" care which is in no way geared to that particular procedure. (Any treatment which was specifically geared to sterilization would evidently amount to formal co-operation.) Concerning advice and information, the same conclusion can be drawn here as in the case of contraception.

Artificial insemination and in vitro fertilization

Artificial insemination consists in the fertilization of a woman's ovum by the introduction of male semen into her body by means other than sexual intercourse. If the semen is that of the woman's own husband we have artificial insemination by husband (AIH), while if it is that of some other man – usually an anonymous donor – we have artificial insemination by donor (AID). Both procedures are normally carried out with the co-operation of nurses.

There is an obvious objection to AID which does not apply to AIH, namely that AID involves the intrusion of a third party into a relationship which we normally conceive as being exclusively between two persons, the married man and woman. By entering into married life together, they have contracted to form an exclusive sexual relationship with each other; and on any reasonable interpretation this exclusive relationship covers not only their sexual acts but also the events which normally result from sexual activity, including the procreation of new life. Catholic moralists have consistently held that this fact alone would be sufficient to rule AID out of consideration. In the recent instruction *Donum Vitae*, for instance, it is argued that

> Respect for the unity of marriage and for conjugal fidelity demands that the child be conceived in marriage; the bond existing between husband and wife accords the spouses, in an objective and inalienable manner, the exclusive right to become father and mother solely through each other. Recourse to the gametes of a third person, in order to have sperm or ovum available, constitutes a violation of the

reciprocal commitment of the spouses and a grave lack in regard to that essential property of marriage which is its unity.[1]

Moreover, the Catholic moral tradition is usually taken to rule out any sort of artificial insemination, AIH just as much as AID. Consider once again the key principle that human sexual activity has both a unitive and a procreative "meaning", and that any attempt to remove either of these meanings from a couple's sexual activity amounts to an attack on a basic human good and is therefore immoral. What this suggests is that human sexual activity and procreation are so closely bound up together that sexual intercourse is not merely the normal way of achieving procreation but the only morally appropriate way of doing so, and that to separate procreation from its grounding in intimate sexual union is to act against the basic human good which is at stake in sexual activity.[2] Are there, in fact, solid grounds for believing that the dissociation of procreation from sexual intercourse is in principle wrong? It will be better to leave this question open for the moment and return to it after we have looked at *in vitro* fertilization, which displays this separation between procreation and the sexual act much more radically than does AIH and AID.

In vitro fertilization (IVF) is a highly complex procedure. It involves a whole team of research scientists, physicians, surgeons and nurses in co-ordinating their several activities so that the different stages of the procedure can all be performed successfully. These stages include prescribing drug treatment for the woman so as to effect superovulation, obtaining ripe ova from her by laparoscopy or some other technique, collecting semen from her partner or a donor, fertilizing the ova *in vitro*, selecting one or more of the resulting embryos for implantation into the woman's uterus and then, finally, carrying out the implantation.

Some troubling questions are raised by the fact that IVF, as currently practised, involves producing large numbers of "spare" embryos, that is, embryos which are not destined for implantation but are eventually discarded, often after having been experimented upon by scientific researchers. These practices of fertilizing human eggs, experimenting upon them and finally destroying them raise the all-important question of the status of the human embryo: is it a human being in the full sense, a

---

[1]. S.C.D.F., Instruction *Donum Vitae*, II, 2. Pope Pius XII had earlier made the same point in his *Discourse to those taking part in the Fourth International Congress of Catholic Doctors*, on 29 September 1949 (*Acta Apostolicae Sedis* 41, 1949).

[2]. See *Donum Vitae*, IIB, 6.

human person? Or is it, on the contrary, a living organism which is only potentially human? If we consider an embryo to be a human person (albeit in an immature state) then we must regard its deliberate destruction as homicide, and we must condemn any and every attempt to experiment upon it as incompatible with its human dignity, unless the experiments are aimed at benefiting that individual human embryo itself. Now just as there is no good reason to deny that the human foetus is a full human being, a person (as we saw in the last chapter), so there is no good reason to deny personhood to the human embryo. The embryo is, of course, a human being in an extremely immature state, its inherent natural capacities and tendencies have only just begun to be unfolded and developed, but these capacities and tendencies do (as far as we can tell) already exist, and will be developed gradually over time. We must once again distinguish between an *immature* human being and a *potential* human being: the human embryo belongs to the first category but not to the second. Hence the deliberate destruction of a human embryo is, morally speaking, an act of the same type as the deliberate killing of a mature human being.[1]

The question "Is IVF a morally acceptable procedure?" must therefore receive a negative answer, on the grounds that at present IVF is in practice inseparable from the widespread deliberate destruction of human embryos. A nurse working in this area would inevitably face difficult problems of co-operation, given that IVF is such a complex business. She would have to ask: "Am I obliged to refuse to co-operate in all IVF

---

[1]   Someone opposing this conclusion may urge that the apparent occurrence of "twinning" in the early embryo renders this view of the matter untenable. For there seem to be occasions when a single human embryo "splits into two", thus giving us identical twins. In this case, the objection would run, one cannot say either that there was a single human being present before the occurrence of "twinning" (for how could one human being become two?) or that there were two human beings present (for the embryo prior to twinning is, to all appearances, in exactly the same condition as one which does not divide). Hence, what we have before twinning takes place is human organic matter which is neither a single human being nor a pair of human beings; personhood is acquired by this matter at some later stage, but is not present in the embryo. However, it can be replied that although the mechanisms responsible for twinning are at present deeply mysterious, it could be that what is present from the beginning is a single human being, and that, at some stage in this embryonic human being's development, and by means of some asexual means of reproduction which we do not understand, a second embryonic human being comes into existence from some of the matter which had previously been part of the first human being. There is no reason for preferring an interpretation of the data which excludes the existence of human persons *ab initio* from one which accepts it.

procedures, or may I co-operate in some of them (e.g., providing ordinary nursing care for a woman before and after her laparoscopy) but not in others (e.g., the laparoscopy itself)?" It would seem unnecessary to examine these problems of co-operation here, because at present IVF is carried out in specialist IVF units in hospitals, and hence there is little chance of a nurse's suddenly and without warning being thrust into such work. The real question for a nurse is whether she should be prepared to choose to work in an IVF unit; and the very nature of this work makes it clear that the answer is No.

Suppose, however, that an IVF unit abandons the practice of fertilizing several ova and resolves to implant all the embryos produced, so that it does not destroy or experiment on embryos. This is sometimes called the "ideal case" of IVF. Would the practice then be morally acceptable, and would a nurse act rightly in participating in the work of the unit? Here we need to consider the fact that even "the ideal case" of IVF involves separating procreation from human sexual activity, as does artificial insemination. Are there grounds for thinking it wrong to bring about this separation?

An important line of argument focuses on the kind of attitude towards a child which is made by one who authorizes and consents to IVF, as well as by those involved in carrying out the procedure. The child is typically regarded as a desired *product*, an object of manufacture, who is produced by the man and woman providing the gametes in co-operation with the IVF team. No longer is the child regarded in the way appropriate to normal human procreation, as a *gift* which supervenes on, and appropriately complements, the act of sexual intimacy which expresses the mutual love and commitment of the parents.[1] In the one case (that of normal procreation through sexual intercourse) the child, considered as a gift which complements the parents' own self-giving in their sexual activity, enters the community of the family as a partner on terms of fundamental

---

[1] The submission of the Catholic bishops' bioethics committee to the Warnock Committee expresses this point as follows:

> ... the IVF child comes into existence, not as a gift supervening on an act expressive of marital union, and so not in the manner of a new partner in the common life so vividly expressed by that act, but rather in the manner of a product of a making (and indeed, typically, as the end-product of a process managed and carried out by persons other than his parents).

(Catholic Bishops' Joint Committee on Bio-Ethical Issues, *In Vitro Fertilisation: Morality and Public Policy*) (Catholic Information Office, Abbots Langley, Herts, 1983), para. 24, p. 14.

equality with his parents. However, in IVF and also in artificial insemination, the child, considered as a product brought into being by his parents in co-operation with the hospital team, is inevitably placed in the relation of product *vis-a-vis* producer, and this is inherently a relation of inequality, of subordination to the power and control of others. This difference of attitudes towards the child is anything but superficial, and it is arguable that to regard a child as "a product of a making" is both wrong in itself and a cause of serious evils in society – even though these evils may not become apparent in the short run. For "the essential conditions of the IVF child's origin... tend to assign this child, in its inception, the same status as other objects of acquisition. The technical skills and decisions of the child's makers will have produced, they hope, a good product, a desirable acquisition. The great evils... of destructive experimentation, observation and selection are also *signs*... of the moral flaw with which we are now concerned: of decisions in which human children are envisaged and conceived as products. For products typically are subject to quality control, utilisation, and discard."[1] Hence, even though a couple may request and participate in IVF from the very best of motives, because they truly want a child and are prepared to devote themselves to the care of that child as parents should, it seems that in choosing that their child be brought into existence in this way they are involving themselves in attitudes and actions which are objectively morally flawed.

On this view, then, a child must be regarded as a gift which complements the mutual self-giving of man and woman as expressed most vividly in sexual intercourse, and which thus enters the family as an equal partner with them. It will follow that any sort of reproductive technique in which the child is treated as a product to be *made* by the use of appropriate techniques will be morally objectionable, and this will apply to artificial insemination (whether AIH or AID) as well as to IVF. The fact that we are dealing here with morally wrong attitudes whose effects in practice may take some time to become obvious may mean that the wrongness of these techniques is perhaps not apparent to many people: this is evidently the case with AIH. If, however, the line of argument sketched here is sound, all these techniques which involve regarding the

---

[1.] *In Vitro Fertilisation: Morality and Public Policy*, para. 27, p. 16. It is regrettable that the Warnock Committee showed no evidence, in their published report, of having considered seriously this argument of the Catholic bishops' committee. I have outlined the argument only in very brief terms here; for a fuller formulation the reader should consult the submission itself.

child as a product brought about by human mastery over raw materials are morally unacceptable. Since, then, AIH and AID, as well as IVF in "the ideal case", are wrong in themselves, formal co-operation in either of them would also be wrong, while material co-operation would be justified only under the same stringent conditions as those specified concerning abortion, contraception and sterilization.

Many of the moral attitudes and convictions which are widespread in the Western world today are so far at odds with Christian and Catholic attitudes that it is to be expected that a Catholic nurse will often find her convictions opposed to those which are taken for granted by her fellow-workers and by patients. But nowhere does this opposition between Christian and non-Christian attitudes seem so obvious and so strong as in the field of sexual ethics. With regard to abortion, Catholic nurses will often find their convictions shared by other people who are non-Catholics or even non-Christians. But the Catholic opposition to contraception and sterilization is not nearly so widely shared by those outside the Church. Hence, with regard to these issues the Catholic nurse is especially liable to feel a kind of isolation from those with whom and among whom she must work. If, then, problems of sexual morality do sometimes arise in the course of her work, it would seem wise for her to give some special reflexion and study to the Church's teaching on them, and thereby to prepare herself – together with the help of prayer – for the decisions which will have to be taken in hospital, or on the health-visiting round, and so on.

★   ★   ★

This Chapter in Summary

The main issues discussed here are those concerning contraception, sterilization, artificial insemination and *in vitro* fertilization. A key principle on which Catholic moralists have relied in discussing these issues is that human sexual activity, rightly viewed, has two essential aspects or "sides" to it: a love-giving or love-expressing or unitive "side", and, on the other hand, a life-bestowing or procreative "side". While it is not easy to prove from neutral premises that the sexual act does have these two "sides" or "meanings", there are certain negative arguments which indicate that this is so. In the case of contraception and sterilization, the fact that the procreation of a new human being is a co-operative activity between a human couple on the one hand and God on the other means that any act of deliberately depriving the sexual act of its procreative effect is an instance of man's unjustly seizing for himself an absolute dominion over human life which does not belong to him. Problems of co-operation which may arise for nurses in these fields have to be resolved in the light of the moral principles governing material co-operation in an evil act. The fact that a child is appropriately regarded as a gift from God and not as the result of skilful human production also indicates that attempts to bypass the sexual act in bringing new human beings into existence are morally wrong; and this applies to both artificial insemination and *in vitro* fertilization. These practices may present problems of co-operation for nurses, although where a procedure is carried out in a specialist clinic, as is IVF, these problems will arise in the first place only if a nurse agrees to work there: clearly she would be unwise to do so.

CHAPTER FOURTEEN

PROFESSIONAL RELATIONSHIPS AND PROFESSIONAL STANDARDS

In this last chapter we return to a topic discussed in Chapter One: the idea of the nurse as a health *professional*, concerned to uphold the standards to which the nursing profession is committed, and concerned also to act with professional integrity and accountability. The fact that nurses are members of a profession gives rise to some ethical problems which call for careful examination. These problems are not, perhaps, as acute and dramatic as those concerning life-and-death issues or honesty and confidentiality, and since they often have to do with a nurse's whole way of thinking about her work, her professional orientation, rather than her response to a given crisis, it would be easy to overlook them. Indeed, many nurses have probably tended to ignore such issues, although this situation may be changing as nurses develop a more lively awareness of the professional character of their work. These problems are considered here under two headings: first, "professional relationships", and secondly, "professional standards".

(1) *Professional Relationships*

By "the nurse's professional relationships" I mean the relationships which she forms, in the course of her work, with other health professionals. The phrase "other health professionals", in turn, covers all the different types of workers engaged professionally in caring for people's health, including nutritionists, physiotherapists and so on. But most ethical problems which come under this general heading will concern nurses in their dealings (1) with other nurses, and (2) with doctors. This section of the present chapter will therefore be particularly concerned with these two types of relationship.

Since all health professionals have the same overriding goal – the restoration and/or maintenance of their patients' health – which calls for a co-ordinated effort from all of them, there are two characteristics which the members of a health-care team should consistently display: first, solidarity with and mutual respect for one another, and secondly, a willingness to co-operate with one another for the good of patients. There are limits to the co-operation which one member of the team can expect from another, especially when there are moral issues at stake; but these attributes of mutual respect and co-operation are nevertheless enormously important. Where they are absent, the well-being of patients may be put at risk. A recent study of professional relationships between general practitioners and nurses in England indicates that at present the ideal of teamwork in primary health-care teams is scarcely realized. According to the survey reported in the study, which examined co-operation between GPs and district nurses, on the one hand, and GPs and health visitors, on the other, only 27 per cent of GP-district nurse pairs worked together properly as a team, and only 11 per cent of GP-health visitor pairs.[1] Clearly this very low level of real teamwork will not be a feature of hospital work, because hospitals are highly-structured institutions in which relationships between professionals are essential to the care of patients. (General practice, by contrast, is a much more open, fluid situation, with less specific goals and less urgency about their achievement.) But it is possible that in many hospitals co-operation between health professionals is not what it should be and that talk about teamwork in nursing, and participation in the hospital team, is not always satisfactorily translated into practice.

Problems involving a nurse and other nurses, on the one hand, and a nurse and one or more doctors, on the other, cannot be resolved except on the basis of a clear idea of the nature of nursing and the nurse's proper role as a health professional. A nurse who misunderstands her own professional role in one of the ways criticized in Chapter One – for example, by regarding herself as wholly devoted to implementing doctors' orders, whatever they might be – will obviously be in no position to handle these nurse-doctor conflicts satisfactorily. More likely than not she will capitulate in the face of the doctor's claims on her obedience, and if his claims are unreasonable, this capitulation could be damaging for the patient and for the nursing staff as a whole – and also for the doctor, because it is not in his real interests, either, for this type of one-sided relationship to hold between himself and nurses.

[1.] A. M. Cartlidge, B. A. Gregson and J. Bond, *The Family Practitioner Services*, (London, 1987).

Two kinds of wrong action can undermine the relationship of respect which should exist between nurses and other health professionals. Both can be described very generally, because they can arise whenever a group of people join together to strive for some common goal – in banking, say, or teaching or agriculture just as much as in nursing or medicine. Suppose X and Y are two people who are required by the nature of their work to co-operate with each other in achieving a common end or goal. Then X can offend against Y through a lack of respect for him or her either:

1. by behaving discourteously, or inconsiderately, or with positive rudeness, to Y; or

2. by failing to give Y that co-operation in advancing their joint goal or goals which Y has a right to expect.

These two types of failure to respect one's professional colleagues will often overlap. For instance, a failure to co-operate as one should with a colleague will usually also amount to an inconsiderate treatment of that colleague. Infringements of duty of these two types may be as common in hospitals and other institutions staffed by nurses as they are in business and industrial workplaces. The ethical problems to which these infringements give rise are difficult because the nurse is faced with a number of obligations which may seem to impel her in contrary directions: concern for the good of her patients, loyalty to her fellow health professionals, loyalty to the institution for which she is working, loyalty to the nursing profession itself, the defence of her own personal integrity and the upholding of the moral principles to which she is committed.

The following report illustrates the first type of lack of respect for one's professional colleagues, since it records one health professional's acting rudely towards another. It was made by a nurse at a hospital in the South of England.

"While working in the antenatal clinic I had to explain methods of care to a patient who was rhesus negative. She had heard of some now-outdated treatments which, she had thought, would be applied to her baby at birth, and while I waited for a doctor to finish with a patient on the other side of the curtain I was reassuring her that these treatments were no longer practised. Having quickly dispensed with his last patient the consultant swept around the curtain and sternly told me not to hold up the clinic by talking to the patient; *he* would tell the patient what she needed to know, he said. This attitude, apart from being pompous, is not for the good of the patient and certainly breaks down any team spirit between doctor and nurse."

This doctor's rudeness was quite unjustified and unprovoked. Insofar as there was any rationale behind his outburst it seems to have been that the nurse was wasting the patient's time, filling her mind with superfluous information, perhaps even confusing and disorientating her. Judging from the report, this does not seem to have been the case. The nurse was, in fact, doing the patient a service in talking to her about the treatment she would probably have to undergo. In general, this sort of explanatory service forms a valuable part of the nurse's work. For, given that the time taken by consultants to describe surgical and other treatments is often inevitably short, the patient needs to have someone at hand who is prepared to explain, in terms which she can readily follow, just what the procedure will amount to and how she is likely to react to it. The nurse has the task of ensuring that the patient has full information about what is to befall her, and, if necessary, of "translating" the consultant's description, which may have been brief and over-technical, into something more easily understood. So the consultant in this situation had no legitimate grounds for complaint against the nurse who was advising the pregnant woman. If this sort of behaviour were a regular practice on his part, the nursing staff could hardly be expected to tolerate it: a complaint should be made to the doctor himself, who should be told that his attitude is unreasonable and offensive in itself, not in the interest of patients, and damaging to good relations between him and nurses.

The following report is an example of the second type of failure to respect one's professional colleagues, that is, a failure to give colleagues the co-operation to which they are entitled. The speaker is a student nurse.

"Sisters often contradict student nurses in front of patients, simply for the sake of some peace and quiet. A patient accused me of not giving him analgesia during the previous night, when, he said, he had been in terrible pain. In fact he had slept soundly all night. He demanded to see 'my superior' so that he could report me. The Sister, when she came, said to him: 'Poor nurse was very tired and couldn't have realised how much pain you were in'. She knew that the man had slept all night, and I felt that her comments had put me in an impossible situation with a patient whom I would have to continue to work with."

Was this nurse's resentment justified? Perhaps it was, because the Sister's remark had confirmed the patient's false belief that she (the nurse) had neglected her duty. Given that the nurse would have to go on nursing this patient, she could hardly fail to worry about what new causes for complaint he might in future try to find in her. Certainly the Sister would seem to have acted wrongly in apparently helping to undermine a patient's trust and confidence in one of her fellow nurses. All the same, one can sympathize with the senior nurse: she may well have thought that the only alternative to saying what she did say would have been to reject the patient's claim that he had been awake and in pain all night; and this might only have increased his irritation and his sense of being hard done by. Was there any other option available to the Sister?

Sometimes a health professional's failure to show respect for his colleagues will be a momentary lapse, perhaps something that happened while he was under strong pressure of various kinds. In this case – and provided that his lapse was a fairly minor one – it could be reasonable for the person witnessing it (or on the receiving end of it) to dismiss it as one of those things that happen all too easily and to take no further action about it. But if we are dealing not with an isolated lapse but with a settled pattern of behaviour, or with a gross failure to respect one's professional colleagues, then the question "Should the matter be taken further?" will arise. This is the problem of when one should "blow the whistle" on one's colleagues by reporting them to higher authority. Clearly this problem arises not only when a nurse is the victim of another health professional's wrong action but also when she witnesses another health professional acting wrongly. Should she try to ensure that some action is taken against the offending health professional? If so, what action?

In theory there should not be much of a problem here. Suppose that the breach of duty is serious enough to call for action, and that the situation cannot be resolved by a private talk between the offending party and the nurse who witnessed his act. Then the nurse should report the incident to her senior nursing officer, or, if the hospital or other institution for which she works has a standard procedure for dealing with such complaints, to the person or body nominated in that procedure. Suppose, for instance, that the act witnessed was one of physical assault of a patient. Here we have an action which is immoral in itself and a clear breach of professional responsibility. The act should, then, be reported to the appropriate person or body so that they can investigate the situation and take whatever disciplinary action is called for.

In practice, however, this line of action may impose such stresses and hardship on a nurse that she may hesitate and even wonder whether it would be wiser to do nothing. She may think this even if it is clear that the offensive behaviour was not a "one-off" occurrence and is likely to recur. One of the most worrying considerations is that the person who is to be reported, and perhaps many of one's fellow nurses, may not take kindly to being treated in this way. Since the nurse who "blows the whistle", unless she simultaneously resigns her position, will have to continue to work in close proximity to the person whom she reports, she will be understandably reluctant to take this step. The unspoken pressure which a nurse will feel not to take any action may be extremely strong. The report *Conscientious Objectors at Work* cites several statements from nurses which testify to the enormous pressure which nurses may be under to say nothing about an incident in which (say) a mentally-ill patient has been physically assaulted. The pressure to conform, and the implied threat that one's life will be made uncomfortable if one speaks out, may come not only from one's fellow nurses on the wards but also from hospital managers, the very people who should ensure that complaints about alleged breaches of conduct are vigorously investigated. One of the testimonies included is from a former psychiatric charge nurse, who said:

> The managers make the right kinds of noises. . . the veil of respectability. The word will get around the institution, and then the normal thing is to make the complainant see the error of his ways. . . That's done in a number of subtle ways, over a drink in the social club, on the wards, little chats: 'You didn't really mean to do this. . .' It starts off normally friendly – then, if the nurse refuses to budge, it's a case of 'discredit the complainant'. You will find commonly, people who have complained in mental hospitals – there will have been very strenuous attempts to find weaknesses in their own character, and use those weaknesses against them. . . And then I've known extremes, like anonymous telephone calls to the person telling them to shut their mouths or else – cars interfered with – and that's the process. . . You'll get personal physical abuse, verbal

abuse, ridicule. I've seen every trick in the book used against nurses who have blown the whistle.[1]

Another report, by a nurse manager at a mental hospital where "a group of staff spoke up about repeated assaults and misuse of patients' money by one of the nurses", indicates the intensity of the pressure on those who took this step:

> They were subject to violence outside: threats were made against them, anonymous phone calls, police had to walk one of them home at night. They were threatened... One of the most serious [incidents] was that one of the girls who was divorced, and living alone with her children, her front door was smashed in in the night. That would be by 'colleagues', if that's the right word to use. They were made to feel uncomfortable.[2]

As the report goes on to say, "Clearly, nurses in some hospitals have real reason to fear reprisals. These can be enough to inhibit all but the bravest – or the most naive – from speaking out."[3] One may also be inhibited from speaking out by a fear of having to go through the investigatory procedure, possibly with several meetings at which one will be interrogated about the grounds of one's complaint. At such meetings one may experience doubt about whether one's claim will be believed, or about whether hospital management will really be prepared to take action against the offender.

In view of these powerful pressures on a nurse to keep quiet, it would seem unreasonable to say that she must always report abuses by fellow health professionals to the appropriate body. Just as it may, under some circumstances, be permissible to co-operate materially in an immoral procedure, so it may be permissible to stand by and make no attempt to stop some abuse which one witnesses from going on. But clearly this will be permissible only when the harm suffered by the individual as a result of speaking up would be so great as to be out of all proportion to the abuse which the patient is suffering. On the other hand, if the abuse amounts to a major violation of the patient's integrity (as it would if it consisted in physical assault or stealing his money, or unreasonably imposing very

---

1. V. Beardshaw, *Conscientious Objectors at Work*, p. 36.
2. *ibid.*, p. 37.
3. *ibid.*

severe limitations on his movements and activity) then the nurse would seem to be morally obliged to act, regardless of the personal consequences for her – even if her taking action would lead to such nastiness being directed against her that she would have to resign her position. It is indeed arguable that sitting back and saying nothing about abuse of patients is itself a type of co-operation in the abuse. For the nurse, as a professional, has a legitimate interest in and responsibility for *everything* that goes on in her working environment: she should regard herself as contributing by her actions to the proper functioning of her hospital or medical practice or health-visiting round, etc., and not merely as being charged with carrying out certain narrowly-circumscribed duties. She cannot, then, maintain that what other health professionals do to their patients is none of her business. The welfare of all the patients is of concern to her, even if she herself nurses only a small number of them. Hence any keeping silent when patients are seriously abused can reasonably be seen as a type of unjust material co-operation in the evil, a connivance with the offending party and against the patient for whom the nurse has a professional responsibility.

(2) *Maintaining professional standards*

The fact that the nurse is a professional means that when she is carrying out her duties in (say) a hospital ward, she acts not simply as an individual but as a representative of a professional body. In her actions she expresses, or should express, the high standards to which her profession is committed. Hence, any failure to carry out her nursing duties will be not only a personal failure on her part but also an act of "letting down" her side, of damaging the profession itself.

A nurse who is alive to the professional character of her work will therefore regard herself not just as an individual possessing nursing skills, or as co-operating with a team of other individuals who happen to share those skills with her, but as representing a whole profession and as expressing in her actions the ideals to which the profession is committed. It follows that her acts should be inspired by respect for her profession, by a desire to see it flourish, and by a concern that its public standing be maintained and enhanced.

Any right action performed by a nurse in the course of her duties will *ipso facto* be an act in which her profession and its standards are respected. So every ethical problem arising for a nurse will be one in which her respect for the profession is at stake. But in the great majority of such problems (as, e.g., those concerning resuscitation, or abortion, or truth-telling, or experimentation on patients) the principal focus of attention will be the rightness or wrongness of the act itself. If the act is wrong, then by performing it the nurse will damage her profession, but the question of professional integrity is secondary here, the question of the moral right-ness or wrongness of the act itself being primary. However, there are some issues in which one's professional integrity, one's success or failure in matching up to the standards of the profession and in promoting the good of the profession as a whole, is (or should be) the primary focus – or, at least, a very important focus – of the nurse's attention when she is trying to decide what to do. There seem to me to be four main types of profession-centred obligation which weigh on nurses, and since all four of them must be stated in general terms, difficulties may arise over how exactly they should be translated into practice. These four general types of obligation are:

(1) The obligation to maintain one's professional knowledge and expertise and to keep abreast of new developments in one's field. This obligation evidently follows from the fact that a professional association is, *inter alia*, the repository of a body of theoretical and practical knowl-edge which is continuously being reviewed and updated in the light of new research. An example of a failure to keep up with important new developments is the ignorance of some older nurses concerning improved means of dealing with pressure areas and sores. As a recent study describes it,

> Even after publication of findings to the contrary, nurses continued to rub soap and water, spirit and a variety of other doubtful applica-tions on patients' skin. For a learner nurse this particular example might pose ethical difficulties. From the college of nursing she will have been supplied with the latest research-based information in relation to the care of pressure areas; yet on the ward she could be told that the sister's policy involves a treatment which the student knows has been shown to be harmful. Given that a nurse is sup-posed to be not only responsible for her actions but also morally accountable for them, this student's choice between following the teachings of the college and obeying the ward sister is a difficult one.[1]

---

1. I. E. Thompson, K. M. Melia and K. M. Boyd, *Nursing Ethics* (Edinburgh, 1983), pp. 53–4.

This problem concerns not only the immediate welfare of the patient but also the nurse's professional integrity, because an up-to-date knowledge of the best treatment of pressure areas and sores is something which should be expected of any nurse, whether she has graduated one or 30 years ago. Would a younger nurse, faced with this problem, be justified in questioning the ward sister's directive and/or lodging a protest about it?

(2) The obligation to bring it about that one's own lifestyle and behaviour conform to the proper image of the nurse as a man or woman of professional integrity. A nurse whose behaviour betrays an indifference to the good of health – by heavy smoking, say, or by a diet centred largely on nutritionally-worthless food – could hardly be regarded as expressing the nursing ideal.[1]

(3) The obligation to take some interest in, and perhaps make some contribution to, deliberations concerning the future direction of the profession. The extent of an individual nurse's obligation in this regard will depend on her own aptitudes and inclinations and the time at her disposal. But some attention to issues such as these is surely required of all nurses by virtue of their professional status. An involvement in these issues could be carried out through a body such as the Royal College of Nursing, and also, in the case of a Catholic nurse, through the local branch of the Catholic Nurses' Guild. Among the particular issues in which one would expect a nurse to take an intelligent interest are: the role of the nurse in the health-care field, especially as compared with that of the doctor; the way in which public resources for health care should be allocated (a concentration of resources on technically-advanced treatment for the acutely ill, or instead, perhaps, a reallocation of resources in favour

---

[1]. A student nurse, writing recently, seizes on this issue concerning diet as a pressing one for nurses:

> As educators, what... is our responsibility to our patients? So often we criticise their lifestyle and, for example, encourage them to stop smoking when they are admitted for treatment of a chest infection. 'Reduce your fat intake – no more chips or fry-ups, drink skimmed milk and change to polyunsaturated fats...'. How often do we give such advice to cardiac patients, but do *we* practise what we preach? Some of the most unhealthy people are nurses; smoking is rife in the profession, and many nurses are seriously overweight! Much of this is caused by conditions of work, canteen food, tempting chocolates in the wards from well-wishing patients and the high stress levels under which we work. The question is, do we have a moral obligation to look after ourselves, as we are the health advocates? (R. Kennedy, contributing to "Moral Matters", in the *Nursing Times*, vol. 84, no. 19, May 11, 1988, p. 49.)

of community health care and preventive medicine?); and the sort of direction in which the health-care system should be going (a more prominent place for private health care and private insurance or a more narrow reliance on state-funded medicine?).

(4) The obligation to reflect on the question of the kinds of industrial action which can be justified. Is it morally right for nurses to go on strike, given that strike action inevitably puts some patients' lives at risk? If so, under what circumstances? If not, could nurses do nothing at all to overcome a situation in which their salaries were unjustly low or their working conditions poor? Does the fact that a nurse is a member of a profession mean that she should never resort to methods of industrial action which the average trade unionist would regard as normal and, indeed, indispensable in pursuit of a just cause?

This issue of industrial action has been much discussed recently, and we may consider it a little more closely here, in order to illustrate the kinds of profession-centred ethical problems which can arise. Some people hold that the nurse's overriding concern for the lives of her patients means that industrial action is out of the question for her, while adding that various other stratagems are available to the profession in its attempt to secure nurses' just demands. (These alternatives include publicity campaigns which appeal to the public's evident respect and affection for nurses.) On the other side, it is claimed that the non-strike options are ineffective and that industrial action should not be ruled out of consideration, provided that adequate emergency services are maintained throughout the strike. This response has been heavily criticized – cogently, it seems to me – on two grounds. First, there are no precise criteria for determining which services are emergency ones and which are not. Even those patients who are not emergency cases are still in a serious enough condition to be in hospital, and their condition may easily deteriorate if they are not provided with consistent and continuing treatment. Secondly, during a strike most hospital wards will be understaffed, and then any sort of unexpected mishap which would ordinarily be noticed and rectified immediately may go unnoticed and unrectified, with, quite possibly, a patient dying as a result. The point here is that hospitals are places where anything can happen at any time, and nurses need to be on hand to deal with the unexpected. In 1987 a woman who was undergoing dialysis at the Western Infirmary in Glasgow bled to death when a tube connecting her to the dialysis machine came loose. At the time the ward was understaffed and there was no nurse present to notice and deal with the mishap: by the time the accident was noticed, it was too late to save the patient's life.[1] Clearly, if nurses go on strike the likelihood of this sort of incident occurring is greatly increased, and no amount of "provision of emergency services" is going to remedy the situation.

The traditional Catholic teaching on the morality of striking can be of use to us here. Consider the following convenient summary of the teaching, which has been developed in such papal encyclicals as Leo XIII's *Rerum Novarum* (1891):

> For a strike to be just, two conditions must be met: the strike may not be a breach of a just labour contract; the strikers may not impose unjust demands. But what is just cannot be narrowly determined... Workers whose wages are below the minimum just wage run no risk of breaching a just labour contract by striking. A contract establishing unjustly low wages is an unjust contract...
>
> [However,] Even though it does not violate justice, a strike may be illicit on other grounds. Since a strike has a twofold effect, the promotion of the workers' interests on the one hand and on the other hand the harmful consequences to the workers and their families, to the employer and his business, and to the public..., charity requires that a strike be undertaken only: (1) when all other feasible methods of settling the dispute have been exhausted, (2) when there is a sound proportion between what the workers hope to gain and the losses and inconveniences that the strike entails, and (3) when there are genuine prospects for a successful outcome... [Moreover,] the strikers are limited to licit means in furthering the strike.[2]

The second of these conditions governing the morality of striking is highly relevant here: there must be "a sound proportion between what

---

1. This incident is reported in the *Nursing Times*, vol. 83, no. 5, February 4, 1987, p. 6 ("Shortages blamed for patient's death"). A hearing at Glasgow Sheriff Court was told that "The number of nurses available at the hospital's renal unit was 'totally inadequate'... Staffing at the hospital had been reduced 'insidiously' since 1980, but the workload had risen fourfold in that time... [The patient] had been very ill after major surgery. She was on a Haemofilter machine 24 hours a day, and the hearing was told that ideally, she should have had a nurse beside her bed virtually all the time." (*ibid.*)

2. L. C. Brown, "Strike", in *The New Catholic Encyclopaedia*, vol. 13, pp. 733–739.

the workers hope to gain and the losses and inconveniences that the strike entails". Given that what is at stake in a nurses' strike is not mere loss of production or financial setbacks but the very lives of human beings, it is difficult to conceive of *any* circumstances in which such a strike would be justified. On this view, recourse to the strike weapon is at odds with the nurse's professional commitment.

So much by way of very brief comment on the sorts of wider social issues raised by the character of modern nursing. Many nurses, unfortunately, still consider problems such as these to be outside their proper concern. But this situation will, it is to be hoped, change as nurses come to realize more and more clearly what it means to be a professional and to have the interests of the profession at heart.

★ ★ ★

This Chapter in Summary

The title of this chapter could cover any and every moral problem arising in nursing practice, but there are some such problems in which the professional character of the nurse's work occupies centre stage, so to speak. This chapter affords only a brief glance at some of these problems. Concerning professional relationships, the question of "blowing the whistle" on one's professional colleagues is liable to produce particularly acute difficulties. Concerning professional standards, there are important questions, of which one – the morality of striking – is given some brief consideration here.

SOME SUGGESTIONS FOR
FURTHER READING

During recent years a number of books and many articles devoted to problems of nursing ethics have appeared, and the choice facing the reader can be bewildering. A glance at T. Pence's *Ethics in Nursing: An Annotated Bibliography* (second edition, New York, 1986) will reveal just how intense a field of study and controversy nursing ethics has become. Many general introductory treatments of nursing ethics are currently available, although most of them have been published in the U.S.A. and are therefore written with the American nursing scene very much in mind. Two recent British publications are I. E. Thompson, K. M. Melia and K. M. Boyd, *Nursing Ethics* (Edinburgh, 1983), and V. Tschudin's *Ethics in Nursing: the Caring Relationship* (London, 1986). These are well worth reading, although they both suffer, in my view, from an insufficiently rigorous consideration of basic issues in general ethical theory. The natural-law ethical tradition has not been well represented in recent nursing ethics books, and has often been outlined and dismissed in a couple of pages (as, for example, in J. L. Muyskens, *Moral Problems in Nursing: A Philosophical Investigation* (Totowa, U.S.A., 1982), pp. 13-14. An exception is E. J. Hayes, P. J. Hayes and D. E. Kelly, *Moral Principles of Nursing* (New York, 1964), but given that this volume appeared so long ago it is inevitably out of date in some respects and also, I believe, largely fails to reveal the real point and underlying rationale of the natural-law ethic. For a more adequate exposition of this moral outlook one should look closely at some of the volumes of Germain Grisez and his philosophical and theological allies, particularly Chapter X and XI of J. M. Boyle, J. M. Finnis and G. G. Grisez, *Nuclear Deterrence and Morality* (Oxford, 1987), as well as J. M. Finnis's *Fundamentals of Ethics* and the volume *Catholic Sexual Ethics* by J. M. Boyle, P. E. Lawler and W. E. May, in which this natural-law ethic is applied to issues of human sexuality. It is only fair to mention, however, that this formulation of natural-law theory on which Grisez and others have been working is not without its critics, such as R. Hittinger in his *A Critique of the New Natural Law Theory* (Notre Dame, U.S.A., 1987). A Catholic approach to bioethical issues is also competently expressed in B. M. Ashley and K. D. O'Rourke, *Ethics of Health Care* (St. Louis, U.S.A., 1986). Given the central importance of the virtues in the moral life, P. T. Geach's *The Virtues* (Cambridge, 1976) could provide a helpful stimulus to discussions in general ethics and its applications. Concerning particular issues of nursing ethics discussed in this book, the Linacre Centre's working party report, *Euthanasia and Clinical Practice*, together with the accompanying study guide (T. Iglesias, *Study Guide to Euthanasia and Clinical Practice* (London, 1984)) will aid reflexion, not only on problems of euthanasia, but on all the life-and-death issues, while in general the case studies assembled in R. M. Veatch's *Case Studies in Nursing Ethics* (Philadelphia, 1987), together with the author's comments, will provide much matter for discussion. For rigorous philosophical argument covering a whole range of crucial bioethical problems the volume *Moral Dilemmas in Modern Medicine*, edited by M. Lockwood (Oxford, 1985) can be recommended. Finally, the periodical *Ethics and Medics*, published monthly by the John XXIII Bioethics Center at Boston, U.S.A., deals briefly but informatively, from the point of view of Catholic moral teaching, with a very wide range of problems in medical and nursing ethics: its very brevity is an asset because the articles often go straight to the heart of the matters being dealt with.

INDEX